FOOD AND BEVERAGE CONSUMPTION AND HEALTH

PORK CONSUMPTION AND HEALTH

FOOD AND BEVERAGE CONSUMPTION AND HEALTH

Additional books and e-books in this series can be found on Nova's website under the Series tab.

FOOD AND BEVERAGE CONSUMPTION AND HEALTH

PORK CONSUMPTION AND HEALTH

FRANK L. MOORE
EDITOR

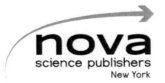

Copyright © 2019 by Nova Science Publishers, Inc.

All rights reserved. No part of this book may be reproduced, stored in a retrieval system or transmitted in any form or by any means: electronic, electrostatic, magnetic, tape, mechanical photocopying, recording or otherwise without the written permission of the Publisher.

We have partnered with Copyright Clearance Center to make it easy for you to obtain permissions to reuse content from this publication. Simply navigate to this publication's page on Nova's website and locate the "Get Permission" button below the title description. This button is linked directly to the title's permission page on copyright.com. Alternatively, you can visit copyright.com and search by title, ISBN, or ISSN.

For further questions about using the service on copyright.com, please contact:
Copyright Clearance Center
Phone: +1-(978) 750-8400   Fax: +1-(978) 750-4470   E-mail: info@copyright.com.

NOTICE TO THE READER

The Publisher has taken reasonable care in the preparation of this book, but makes no expressed or implied warranty of any kind and assumes no responsibility for any errors or omissions. No liability is assumed for incidental or consequential damages in connection with or arising out of information contained in this book. The Publisher shall not be liable for any special, consequential, or exemplary damages resulting, in whole or in part, from the readers' use of, or reliance upon, this material. Any parts of this book based on government reports are so indicated and copyright is claimed for those parts to the extent applicable to compilations of such works.

Independent verification should be sought for any data, advice or recommendations contained in this book. In addition, no responsibility is assumed by the Publisher for any injury and/or damage to persons or property arising from any methods, products, instructions, ideas or otherwise contained in this publication.

This publication is designed to provide accurate and authoritative information with regard to the subject matter covered herein. It is sold with the clear understanding that the Publisher is not engaged in rendering legal or any other professional services. If legal or any other expert assistance is required, the services of a competent person should be sought. FROM A DECLARATION OF PARTICIPANTS JOINTLY ADOPTED BY A COMMITTEE OF THE AMERICAN BAR ASSOCIATION AND A COMMITTEE OF PUBLISHERS.

Additional color graphics may be available in the e-book version of this book.

Library of Congress Cataloging-in-Publication Data

ISBN: 978-1-53614-991-3

Published by Nova Science Publishers, Inc. † *New York*

CONTENTS

Preface		vii
Chapter 1	Macro- and Micromineral Contents in Raw and Cooked Pork Meat and Pig Edible Offal *Vladimir Tomović, Mila Tomović, Branislav Šojić, Marija Jokanović and Snežana Škaljac*	1
Chapter 2	Pork Foodborne Parasites of Public Health Interest in Mexico *I. B. Hernandez-Cortazar, E. Guzman-Marin, K. Y. Acosta-Viana, A. Ortega-Pacheco, J. I. Chan-Perez and M. Jimenez-Coello*	45
Chapter 3	Pork Meat Consumption and Salmonellosis Incidence in European Countries: An Ecologic Study *Alberto Arnedo-Pena and M. Rosario Pac-Sa*	79
Index		113

PREFACE

In this compilation, the authors provide an overview of the existing literature on the content of nine most abundant minerals (potassium – K, phosphorous – P, sodium – Na, magnesium – Mg, calcium – Ca, zinc – Zn, iron – Fe, copper – Cu and manganese – Mn) in major raw and cooked pork meat cuts.

The ingestion of raw or undercooked pork poses a public health risk, since pork is the main transmitter of parasites, which include the protozoa *Toxoplasma gondii* and the helminths *Trichinella spiralis* and *Taenia solium*. These three 'T' porkborne parasites have been responsible for most of the porkborne illnesses throughout history, and they are still endemic and therefore an important public-health concern.

In the concluding study, Spearman's correlation coefficient was used to study the relationship salmonellosis and explanatory variables. Second, a multilevel linear regression analysis was carried out with two levels: region, occidental and oriental, European countries, and climate. Additionally, Stata ®14 version was used in the statistical analysis.

Chapter 1 - Meat is one of the most nutritious foods that humans can consume, and is defined as the flesh (skeletal muscles) of animals used as food. In addition to protein and fat, meat is a significant source of several micronutrients (minerals and vitamins). Edible offal is also a form of meat which is used as food, but which is not skeletal muscles, and in general possesses higher contents of some micronutrients, especially minerals and vitamins, than muscular tissue. Minerals are the inorganic elements other than carbon, hydrogen, oxygen and nitrogen, which remain behind in the ash when food is incinerated. They are usually divided into two groups – macrominerals (main elements) and microminerals (trace elements) or into three groups – main elements (macrominerals), trace elements (microminerals) and ultra-trace elements. Data on the mineral composition of the raw and cooked pork meat and pig edible offal are available in numerous research papers, food composition tables and databases. The aim of this chapter is to provide an overview of the existing literature on the content of nine most abundant minerals (potassium – K, phosphorous – P, sodium – Na, magnesium – Mg, calcium – Ca, zinc – Zn, iron – Fe, copper – Cu and manganese – Mn) in the major raw and cooked pork meat cuts (tenderloin, ham, loin and shoulder) and pig edible offal (tongue, heart, lungs, liver, spleen, kidney, brain and spinal cord). The mineral levels in raw pork meat and pig edible offal are variable, ranging from 150 to 480 mg/100g for potassium; 139 to 502.0 mg/100g for phosphorous; 38.11 to 190 mg/100g for sodium; 8.3 to 34 mg/100g for magnesium; 3.8 to 35 mg/100g for calcium; 0.67 to 10.1 mg/100g for zinc; 0.46 to 45.59 mg/100g for iron; 0.039 to 2.7 mg/100g for copper; and from 0.0038 to 0.390 mg/100g for manganese. Changes in the mineral content usually occur in the processing of raw animal materials, e.g., in thermal processes and material separations. Generally, most cooked pork meat cuts and pig edible offal contain minerals, except potassium and sodium, at or above the levels in the raw tissues. Potassium and sodium tend to markedly decrease during cooking.

Chapter 2 - The ingestion of raw or undercooked pork poses a public health risk, since pork is the main transmitter of parasites, which include the protozoa *Toxoplasma gondii* (*T. gondii*) and the helminths *Trichinella spiralis* (*T. spiralis*) and *Taenia solium* (*T. solium*). These three 'T' porkborne parasites have been responsible for most of the porkborne illnesses throughout history; they are still endemic, and therefore are important public-health concerns, in developing countries. In Mexico, these three 'T' porkborne parasites are considered re-emerging parasites, and they represents a risk for the population that consumes large quantities of pork. Currently, inspection procedures are effective in eliminating the majority of the risks from *T. spiralis* and *T. solium* in certified slaughterhouses, due to the training of inspectors in the detection of tissue cysts. However, there are still clandestine slaughterhouses that do not have adequate surveillance methods to identify these parasites. Furthermore, for *T. gondii* no suitable methods for post-slaughter detection are available, where intervention measures at the animal level may be key to successful prevention. Early detection of the parasite is not easy, and the implementation of molecular techniques must be improved and made available mainly in endemic areas, in order to establish an accurate diagnosis, because isolation procedures are long, more expensive and often not sufficiently sensitive. The objectives of this chapter are to describe the epidemiological situation of these three parasites transmitted by pork in Mexico, outline the main lines of prevention, and describe the molecular methods that can be used for the early and accurate detection.

Chapter 3 - *Introduction:* In European countries salmonellosis incidence is elevated and it is generally associated with the consumption of eggs, eggs-products and poultry meat, while *S.* Enteritidis is the more reported serotype. However, the incidence of *S* Typhimurium salmonellosis with its monophasic variant is increasing, and swine is considered as an important reservoir of *S.* Typhimurium. The authors' hypothesis is that pork meat consumption in European countries may be associated with salmonellosis incidence. *Material and methods:* The average salmonellosis incidence rate in 31 European countries during the period 2013-2014 was obtained from European Centre for Disease Prevention and Control and European Food Safety Authority. Consumption of pork meat, bovine meat, poultry and eggs in these countries during 2013 was retrieved from the Food and Agriculture Organization. Socioeconomic, demographic, health organization and climate variables were taken from different sources in order to adjust the statistical models. First, Spearman's correlation coefficient was used to study the relationship salmonellosis and explanatory variables. Second, a multilevel linear regression analysis was carried out with two levels: region, occidental and oriental, European countries, and climate (Mediterranean,

Atlantic, continental, and sub-arctic). Stata ®14 version was used in the statistical analysis. *Results:* In the period, the average of salmonellosis incidence rate was 19.1 cases per 100,000 inhabitants (range 2.05-109.6), and the median of pork meat consumption was 34.96 kg/capita/year (range 21.01-52.56). In the multilevel model, salmonellosis incidence increases by 0.79 (95% CI [confidence interval] 0.11-1.48; p = 0.023) with the increase in pork meat consumption, adjusted by GINI index, -2.75 (95% CI -4.20- -1.30; p = 0.000). Egg consumption had no significant association with salmonellosis, (1.69 95% CI -0.70-4.07 p = 0.165). In addition a dose-response pork meat consumption and salmonellosis was found (p = 0.001). The interclass correlation coefficient was 0.31 (95% CI 0.04-0.83), the proportion of total salmonellosis variance among countries. The models presented acceptable goodness of fit tests. Limitations of this study include its ecological approach, national differences in salmonellosis report and control, no distinction of *Salmonella* outbreaks, and no differentiation among *Salmonella* serotypes. *Conclusion:* The authors' study suggests that pork meat consumption is associated with salmonellosis incidence in European countries. An increment and optimization of control and prevention measures in the farm-to-consumption chain for pork products are recommended.

In: Pork Consumption and Health
Editor: Frank L. Moore

ISBN: 978-1-53614-991-3
© 2019 Nova Science Publishers, Inc.

Chapter 1

MACRO- AND MICROMINERAL CONTENTS IN RAW AND COOKED PORK MEAT AND PIG EDIBLE OFFAL

Vladimir Tomović[1,*], Mila Tomović[2], Branislav Šojić[1], Marija Jokanović[1] and Snežana Škaljac[1]

[1]University of Novi Sad, Faculty of Technology Novi Sad, Novi Sad, Serbia
[2]Technical School "Pavle Savić," Novi Sad, Serbia

ABSTRACT

Meat is one of the most nutritious foods that humans can consume, and is defined as the flesh (skeletal muscles) of animals used as food. In addition to protein and fat, meat is a significant source of several micronutrients (minerals and vitamins). Edible offal is also a form of meat which is used as food, but which is not skeletal muscles, and in general possesses higher contents of some micronutrients, especially minerals and vitamins, than muscular tissue. Minerals are the inorganic elements other than carbon, hydrogen, oxygen and nitrogen, which remain behind in the

---

* Corresponding Author E-mail: tomovic@uns.ac.rs.

ash when food is incinerated. They are usually divided into two groups – macrominerals (main elements) and microminerals (trace elements) or into three groups – main elements (macrominerals), trace elements (microminerals) and ultra-trace elements. Data on the mineral composition of the raw and cooked pork meat and pig edible offal are available in numerous research papers, food composition tables and databases. The aim of this chapter is to provide an overview of the existing literature on the content of nine most abundant minerals (potassium – K, phosphorous – P, sodium – Na, magnesium – Mg, calcium – Ca, zinc – Zn, iron – Fe, copper – Cu and manganese – Mn) in the major raw and cooked pork meat cuts (tenderloin, ham, loin and shoulder) and pig edible offal (tongue, heart, lungs, liver, spleen, kidney, brain and spinal cord). The mineral levels in raw pork meat and pig edible offal are variable, ranging from 150 to 480 mg/100g for potassium; 139 to 502.0 mg/100g for phosphorous; 38.11 to 190 mg/100g for sodium; 8.3 to 34 mg/100g for magnesium; 3.8 to 35 mg/100g for calcium; 0.67 to 10.1 mg/100g for zinc; 0.46 to 45.59 mg/100g for iron; 0.039 to 2.7 mg/100g for copper; and from 0.0038 to 0.390 mg/100g for manganese. Changes in the mineral content usually occur in the processing of raw animal materials, e.g., in thermal processes and material separations. Generally, most cooked pork meat cuts and pig edible offal contain minerals, except potassium and sodium, at or above the levels in the raw tissues. Potassium and sodium tend to markedly decrease during cooking.

Keywords: minerals, pork meat, pig edible offal

MINERALS

Minerals are the inorganic elements other than carbon, hydrogen, oxygen and nitrogen, which remain behind in the ash when food is incinerated. They are usually divided into two groups – macrominerals (main elements) and microminerals (trace elements) or into three groups – main elements (macrominerals), trace elements (microminerals) and ultra-trace elements. Many of minerals are essential for plants, animals and humans. The main elements (Na, K, Ca, Mg, Cl, P, S) are essential for human beings in amounts >50 mg/day. Trace elements (Fe, I, F, Zn, Se, Cu, Mn, Cr, Mo, Co, Ni) are essential in contents of <50 mg/day. Ultra-trace elements are: Al, As, Ba, Bi, B, Br, Cd, Cs, Ge, Hg, Li, Pb, Rb, Sb, Si, Sm,

Sn, Sr, Tl, Ti and W (Reilly, 2002; Belitz et al., 2009). Minerals have very varied functions (electrolytes, enzyme constituents, building materials in bones and teeth) in the human body and they must be obtained from diet because they cannot be synthesized. Main functions of minerals in the human body are shown in Table 1 (The National Academy of Sciences, The Health and Medicine Division, USA, 2018).

Dietary reference intake (DRI) is the general term for a set of reference values used to plan and assess nutrient intakes of healthy people. Health authorities in most countries have established recommendations for daily intake levels of essential minerals. DRI of nutrients vary by age and gender. DRI for minerals (K, P, Na, Mg, Ca, Zn, Fe, Cu and Mn) recommended by The National Academies (The National Academy of Sciences, The Health and Medicine Division, USA, 2018) are shown in Table 2.

The Reference Daily Intake (RDI) is used to determine the Daily Value (DV) of foods, which is printed on nutrition facts labels (as % DV). DVs were developed by the U.S. Food and Drug Administration (U.S. FDA, 2000) to help consumers determine the level of various nutrients in a standard serving of food in relation to their approximate requirement for it (Table 3).

Table 1. Main functions of minerals in the human body

Mineral	Function
K	Maintains fluid volume inside/outside of cells and thus normal cell function; acts to blunt the rise of blood pressure in response to excess sodium intake, and decrease markers of bone turnover and recurrence of kidney stones
P	Maintenance of pH, storage and transfer of energy and nucleotide synthesis
Na	Maintains fluid volume outside of cells and thus normal cell function
Mg	Cofactor for enzyme systems
Ca	Essential role in blood clotting, muscle contraction, nerve transmission, and bone and tooth formation
Zn	Component of multiple enzymes and proteins; involved in the regulation of gene expression
Fe	Component of haemoglobin and numerous enzymes; prevents microcytic hypochromic anaemia
Cu	Component of enzymes in iron metabolism
Mn	Involved in the formation of bone, as well as in enzymes involved in amino acid, cholesterol, and carbohydrate metabolism

Table 2. Dietary reference intake for minerals

Life stage group	K (mg/d)	P (mg/d)	Na (mg/d)	Mg (mg/d)	Ca (mg/d)	Zn (mg/d)	Fe (mg/d)	Cu (mg/d)	Mn (mg/d)
I: 0–6 months	400	100	120	30	200	2	0.27	0.20	0.003
I: 7–12 months	700	275	370	75	260	3	11	0.22	0.6
C: 1–3 years	3000	460	1000	80	700	3	7	0.34	1.2
C: 4–8 years	3800	500	1200	130	1000	5	10	0.44	1.5
M/F: 9–13 years	4500	1250	1500	240	1300	8	8	0.70	1.9/1.6
M/F: 14–18 years	4700	1250	1500	410/360	1300	11/9	11/15	0.89	2.2/1.6
M/F: 19–30 years	4700	700	1500	400/310	1000	11/8	8/18	0.90	2.3/1.8
M/F: 31–50 years	4700	700	1500	420/320	1000	11/8	8/18	0.90	2.3/1.8
M/F: 51–70 years	4700	700	1300	420/320	1000/1200	11/8	8/8	0.90	2.3/1.8
M/F: >70 years	4700	700	1200	420/320	1200	11/8	8/8	0.90	2.3/1.8
P: 14–18 years	4700	–	1500	–	1300	–	–	–	–
P: 19–50 years	4000	–	1500	–	1000	–	–	–	–
P: ≤18 years	–	1250	–	400	–	12	27	1.00	2.0
P: 19–30 years	–	700	–	350	–	11	27	1.00	2.0
P: 31–50 years	–	700	–	360	–	11	27	1.00	2.0
L: 14–18 years	5100	–	1500	–	1300	–	–	–	–
L: 19–50 years	5100	–	1500	–	1000	–	–	–	–
L: ≤18 years	–	1250	–	360	–	13	10	1.30	2.6
L: 19–30 years	–	700	–	310	–	12	9	1.30	2.6
L: 31–50 years	–	700	–	320	–	12	9	1.30	2.6

mg/d – milligram/day; I – infants; C – children; M/F – males/females; P – pregnancy; L – lactation.

Macro- and Micromineral Contents in Raw ...

Table 3. Reference daily intake for minerals (mg)

K	P	Na	Mg	Ca	Zn	Fe	Cu	Mn
Daily values for infants								
–	500	–	70	600	5.0	15	0.6	–
Daily values for children less than 4 years of age								
–	800	–	200	800	8.0	10	1.0	–
Daily values for adults and children 4 or more years of age								
3500	1000	2400	400	1000	15	18	2.0	2.0
Daily values for pregnant and lactating women								
–	1300	–	450	1300	15	18	2.0	–

mg – milligram.

The importance of minerals as food ingredients depends not only on their nutritional and physiological roles. They contribute to food flavour and activate or inhibit enzyme-catalysed and other reactions, and they affect the colour and texture of food (Belitz et al., 2009).

PORK MEAT

In living animals, muscles are essential for maintaining the shape of the body in a particular position. Even standing still requires muscular activity. Without normal muscle tone, as during sleep or anaesthesia, maintenance of posture is not possible. Muscles also enable the body of an animal to bend and systematically move and change the support of its limbs, and thereby altering its relation to its environment. Such movement, when suitably coordinated, results in specific actions such as locomotion. Both posture and movement are basic to the survival of an animal (Davies, 2004). There are two general types of muscle – striated and smooth – with this nomenclature derived from the microscopic appearance. Striated muscle has striations while smooth does not. Striated muscle can be further subdivided into skeletal and cardiac. Skeletal muscle, as the name implies, is generally attached to the skeleton. It contains the other tissue types (nerve, epithelia, connective tissue) to a much lesser extent than other tissues and organ systems. Skeletal muscle is the single largest organ mass in the vertebrate body (Swartz, et al., 2009).

The conversion of muscle to meat is a complex process involving many biochemical and physical changes. Muscle tissue is converted from an extensible, metabolically active system to one that is inextensible and quiescent in regard to its biochemical reactions. The speed and extent of *post-mortem* metabolism has a profound effect on the properties of the muscle and its subsequent use for food (Greaser, 2001).

Consumption of meat is generally synonymous with human development. Meat is one of the most nutritious foods that humans can consume, and is defined as the flesh (skeletal muscles) of animals used as food (Jensen et al., 2004; Lawrie and Ledward, 2006). Red meat includes beef, veal, pork and lamb (fresh, minced and frozen) (Williamson et al., 2005). Pork meat is the most widely consumed meat in the world, and the consumption has been steadily increasing (Williamson et al., 2005; FAOSTAT, 2018).

Pork meat quality is known to be influenced by a number of *pre-* and *post-mortem* factor. Quality of pork primary depend on multiple interactive effects of genotype (genetic background, presence of unfavourable alleles at the major genes hal and RN^-), rearing conditions (feeding level, housing and environmental conditions, production system), pre-slaughter handling, and carcass and meat processing (Rosenvold and Andersen, 2003; Olsson and Pickova, 2005).

Meat quality has six dimensions: nutritional quality, sensory quality, technological quality, hygienic quality, toxicological quality and immaterial quality. The nutritive factors of meat quality include proteins and their composition, fats and their composition, micronutrients (minerals and vitamins), utilisation, digestibility and biological value (Honikel, 1999; Olsson and Pickova, 2005).

In a broad sense the composition of meat can be approximated to 75% of water, 19% of protein, 3.5% of soluble, non-protein, substances and 2.5% of fat (Lawrie and Ledward, 2006). In addition to protein and fat, meat is a significant source of several micronutrients (minerals and vitamins).

The nutrient levels in foods are variable. The major sources of variability in nutrient composition are the wide diversity of soil and climatic conditions (geographical origin), seasonal variations, physiological state and maturity, as well as cultivar and breed (Greenfield and Southgate, 2003). The continuous innovations in the breeding systems, rearing practices, feeds composition, changes in slaughtering methods and ageing, largely contribute to induced changes in the content of some of micronutrients in meat (Lombardi-Boccia et al., 2005; Greenfield et al., 2009). According to Hermida et al., (2006), the average mineral contents in tissue depend, in part, on the type of cut (anatomical location of a muscle, i.e., its function in the body), the age of the animal and various other factors. Greenfield and Southgate (2003) concluded that the major sources of variation in animal products are the proportion of lean to fat tissue, and the proportion of edible to inedible materials (bone and gristle). Variations in the lean-fat ratio affect the levels of most nutrients, which are distributed differently in the two fractions.

PIG EDIBLE OFFAL

Animal by-products, or offal, include all parts of a live animal that are not part of the dressed carcass. Noncarcass material such as skin, blood, bones, meat trimmings, fatty tissues, feet, and internal organs of slaughtered pigs contribute to a wide variety of products including human or pet food or processed materials in animal feed, fertilizer or fuel (Toldrá et al., 2012). In general, the total by-products range from 10 to 30% of the live weight of pig (Ockerman and Basu, 2004).

Animal by-products fall into two categories and the divisions are edible and inedible. Biologically, most noncarcass material is edible if the product is cleaned, handled and processed appropriately. The yield of edible by-products from pig varies tremendously depending on sex, live weight, fatness and methods of collection (Ockerman and Basu, 2004).

Edible by-products can be categorized into edible organs, glands, and edible fats (Spooncer, 1988; Ockerman and Basu, 2004). Edible offal, sometimes called "variety meat" or "fancy meat," include the liver, heart, kidney, tongue and other products (other organs, intestines and stomach) frequently used as edible by-products (Ockerman and Basu, 2004). Therefore, edible offal is also a form of meat which is used as food, but which is not skeletal muscles. According to Serbian Regulation (1985), the edible offal of a slaughtered pig, removed during carcass dressing, includes: tongue, heart, lungs, liver, spleen, kidney, brain, spinal cord, testicles, blood, part of the stomach and colon and intestines.

While muscle foods are the more commonly consumed portion of animal, edible by-products such as the entrails and internal organs are also widely consumed (Toldrá et al., 2012). What is considered edible in one region may be considered inedible in another. Many factors influence the consumption of edible offal such as custom, religion, palatability and reputation. Edible offal are often different from skeletal tissue in structure, composition, functional and sensory properties (Spooncer, 1988; Ockerman and Basu, 2004). In general, they have a good nutritional value due to the high protein and low fat levels as well as good content in minerals and vitamins (Nollet and Toldrá, 2011).

Edible by-products from pig slaughter are part of the diet in different countries worldwide (Nollet and Toldrá, 2011), as a component of kitchen-style food preparations or as processed meat products (Ockerman and Basu 2004; Toldrá et al., 2012). The structure of the edible offal clearly influences the possible uses of these products. Brains are usually prepared for the table rather than for use in manufactured meat products. Because of soft texture, brains are blanched to firm the tissue before proceeding with other cooking methods. Hearts are used as table meats. Whole heart can be stuffed in a variety of ways and roasted or braised. Sliced heart meat is grilled or sautéd. Heart meat is also used in sausages and manufactured meats. Kidney are used whole or sliced, and generally either grilled, sautéd or braised, but they are not used to any extent in manufactured meat products. Liver is the most widely used edible offal and is used in many types of manufactured meat products. Livers from pigs are better suited to manufactured meats, particularly liver sausages paté because they have a strong flavour. Pig lungs are mainly used to make stuffing and some types of sausages and manufactured meat. They have limited other uses but may be braised either whole or cubed. Spleens are minced and used in stuffings or manufactured meats. Tongues are used fresh or salted and generally boiled or braised, as well as may be canned (Ognjanović et al., 1985; Spooncer, 1988).

Fat, total fat, crude fat and total lipids are all terms covering more or less the same components (Leth, 2004). There are four sources of lipid in meat animals: the muscle fibres, subcutaneous adipose tissue, intramuscular adipose tissue and abdominal adipose tissue (Smith et al., 2004). In many countries, fat is an unpopular constituent of meat animals for consumers, being considered unhealthy. Yet fat and fatty acids, whether in adipose tissue or muscle, contribute importantly to various aspects of animal tissue quality and are central to the nutritional value of animal tissue (Wood et al., 2008).

Edible animal tissues (meat and offal) are not only the elementary sources of nutrients, but may also contain chemical substances with toxic properties (Dabrowski, 2004). Many of the toxic chemicals are efficiently retained in the edible offal, especially in liver and kidney (Dabrowski and Zdzislaw, 2004; Tomović et al., 2011a, c; 2013a; 2016c; Jokanović et al., 2013).

MINERAL CONTENTS OF RAW PORK MEAT

Corresponding data for the mineral (K, P, Na, Mg, Ca, Zn, Fe, Cu and Mn) contents of the major skeletal muscles/muscle groups (tenderloin, ham, loin and shoulder) from the commercial and indigenous pigs are shown in Table 4 and Table 5. These muscles/muscle groups represent the main muscle mass (main raw pork meat cuts) of a pig. Among the skeletal muscle tissues (muscle groups – raw pork meat cuts), potassium is the most abundant mineral, followed by phosphorous, sodium, magnesium, calcium, zinc, iron, copper and manganese. Overall, there are large variations in the

Table 4. Mineral contents (mg/100g) of raw pork meat from the commercial pigs

Source	Muscle/muscle group	K	P	Na	Mg	Ca	Zn	Fe	Cu	Mn
Australia – Greenfield et al., (2009)	Fillet, lean	390	–	43	26	3.8	1.75	0.86	0.082	0.0105
	Topside steak, lean	370	–	48	25	4.3	1.50	0.73	0.061	0.0086
	Loin steak/medallion, lean	420	–	46	27	5.6	1.55	0.54	0.039	0.0053
Denmark – Danish Food Composition Database (2018)	Tenderloin, trimmed	480	220	100	25.3	8.00	1.83	1.02	0.100	0.014
	Ham, topside (SM), lean	387	209	42.4	25.2	4.24	3.57	0.463	0.100	0.007
	Loin, lean	400	195	83.0	26.0	7.00	3.60	0.710	0.100	0.013
Finland – Fineli - Finnish Food Composition Database (2018)	Fillet, sirloin	280.0	160.0	42.0	20.0	7.4	1.8	0.6	–	–
	Shoulder	320.0	180.0	69.0	21.0	8.0	2.8	1.1	–	–
Italy – Food Composition Database for Epidemiological Studies in Italy (2015)	Leg, lean, wsb	370	233	76	17	12	2.40	1.6	0.15	trace
	Leg, heavy, wsb	370	176	76	17	8	2.40	1.7	0.15	0.01
	Lombo, light, wsb	220	150	73	24	7	1.80	1.3	0.15	0.01
	Lombo, heavy, wsb	300	158	59	17	7	1.80	1.4	0.15	trace
	Shoulder, light, wsb	210	180	73	24	7	1.80	1.2	0.15	0.02
	Shoulder, heavy, wsb	150	150	73	17	6	1.80	1.2	0.15	trace
Lawrie and Ledward (2006)	Pork	400	223	45	26.1	4.3	2.4	1.4	0.1	–
Norway – The Norwegian Food Composition Table (2018)	Tenderloin	408	211	44	26	5	2	1.3	0.08	–
	Inside round	393	226	44	26	4	1.8	0.9	0.06	–
	Striploin	400	219	41	27	4	1.4	0.8	0.04	–
	Shoulder	377	204	52	23	4	2.7	1.3	0.08	–

Table 5. Mineral contents (mg/100g) of raw pork meat from the indigenous pigs

Source	Pig genotype	Rearing system	Live weight (kg)	Muscle/ muscle group	K	P	Na	Mg	Ca	Zn	Fe	Cu	Mn
Galián et al., (2007)	CM	C	138.2	LL	310.44	198.84	40.59	19.22	5.21	2.18	4.61	0.42	–
	CMxIB	C	141.8		327.21	200.26	44.33	22.36	5.66	2.16	8.15	0.55	–
Galián et al., (2009)	CM	O	>125	LL	351.0	206.0	46.7	24.1	5.9	1.4	3.0	0.2	–
			<125		367.8	211.1	50.8	25.0	6.4	1.5	2.7	0.2	–
		I	>125	LL	309.6	197.8	42.4	19.6	5.3	2.1	4.3	0.4	–
			<125		336.1	196.2	58.3	23.1	6.7	1.8	3.5	0.3	–
Poto et al., (2007)	CM	O	110	LL	349.33	205.4	39.98	21.99	5.48	1.43	4.30	0.37	–
	CMxIB				364.41	214.73	46.41	23.56	5.55	1.70	5.87	0.59	–
	CMxLW				351.56	208.39	38.11	22.10	4.61	1.49	5.68	0.44	–
Tomović et al., (2014a)	SBM	FR	up to 150	PM	421.7	216.8	61.3	25.1	5.98	2.89	2.45	0.170	0.022
				SM	380.4	219.4	80.0	24.1	8.27	2.51	1.95	0.143	0.021
				LD	376.7	201.1	55.9	22.4	6.00	2.15	1.35	0.098	0.017
				TB	393.7	197.7	65.1	24.2	6.81	3.83	1.64	0.140	0.021
Tomović et al., (2016a)	SBM	C	up to 100	PM	303	228	58.4	22.8	7.38	3.25	2.74	0.15	–
				SM	297	224	53.1	24.7	7.68	3.47	1.85	0.11	–
				LTL	296	224	50.3	23.5	5.46	2.35	1.08	0.10	–
				TB	286	218	59.2	22.6	6.22	3.90	3.26	0.14	–
Tomović et al., (2016b)	WM	C	up to 150	LL	291	218	45.1	19.3	7.92	1.84	0.94	0.063	0.0082
	DWM				298	226	42.2	19.5	6.24	1.64	0.55	0.050	0.0059

Source	Muscle/muscle group	K	P	Na	Mg	Ca	Zn	Fe	Cu	Mn
USA – USDA Food Composition Databases (2018)	Loin, tenderloin, slo	399	247	53	27	5	1.89	0.98	–	–
	Heg (ham), whole, slo	369	229	55	25	6	2.27	1.01	–	–
	Loin, whole, slo	389	211	52	23	17	1.84	0.84	–	–
	Shoulder, whole, slo	341	202	76	21	14	3.14	1.22	–	–
Slovak Republic – Slovak Food Composition Database (2018)	Tenderloin	359	222	49	25	5	1.99	1.2	–	–
	Leg	162	161	75	23	17	2.84	1.74	0.08	–
	Loin	220	139	76	20	15	1.6	2.38	0.14	–
	Shoulder	242	167	74	23	14	2.61	2.06	–	–
Republic of Serbia – Tomović et al., (2011b); average of 10 genotypes	SM	280	225	59.8	26.6	11.8	2.70	1.42	0.32	0.025
Republic of Serbia – Tomović et al., (2015b,c); average of 5 purebreds	SM	285	227	62.2	26.9	12.0	2.72	1.48	0.31	0.26
	LTL	280	222	59.1	26.4	11.6	2.75	1.36	0.32	0.24
Republic of Serbia – Tomović et al., (2016b)	LL	348	233	44.7	19.4	6.22	1.35	0.46	0.043	0.0058

SM – *M. semimembranosus*; wsb – without visible fat; slo – separable lean only; LTL – *M. longissimus thoracis et lumborum*; LL – *M. longissimus lumborum*.

Source	Pig genotype	Rearing system	Live weight (kg)	Muscle/ muscle group	K	P	Na	Mg	Ca	Zn	Fe	Cu	Mn
Despotović et al., (2018b, in press)	WM (DWM) WM	C	up to 180	LL	334	228	40.2	25.4	5.85	1.79	0.73	0.064	0.0061
					339	227	41.4	25.4	6.16	1.68	0.63	0.043	0.0038
Tomović et al., (2016c)	BS	SO	up to 130	Loin	339	198	50.6	27.8	7.10	3.06	2.07	0.099	0.020
				Ham	346	206	58.4	28.5	7.00	4.66	2.69	0.137	0.024
				Shoulder	316	181	60.7	25.0	7.77	5.43	2.76	0.150	0.025
				Neck	267	159	58.8	21.7	6.91	5.19	2.36	0.120	0.020

CM – Chato Murciano; IB – Iberian; LW – Large White; SBM – Swallow-Belly Mangalica; C – commercial; O – outdoor; I – indoor; FR – free-range; LL – *M. longissimus lumborum*; PM – *M. psoas major*; SM – *M. semimembranosus*; LD – *M. longissimus dorsi*; TB – *M. triceps brachii*; LTL – *M. longissimus thoracis et lumborum*; WM – White Mangalica; D – Duroc; BS – Black Slavonian; SO – semi-outdoor; LL – *M. longissimus lumborum*.

mineral contents of pork meat, ranging from 150 to 480 mg/100g for potassium; 139 to 247 mg/100g for phosphorous; 38.11 to 100 mg/100g for sodium; 17 to 28.5 mg/100g for magnesium; 3.8 to 17 mg/100g for calcium; 1.35 to 5.43 mg/100g for zinc; 0.46 to 8.15 mg/100g for iron; 0.039 to 0.59 mg/100g for copper; and from 0.0038 to 0.26 mg/100g for manganese. For a number of items listed, no values for manganese were available.

MINERAL CONTENTS OF RAW PIG EDIBLE OFFAL

Corresponding data for the mineral (K, P, Na, Mg, Ca, Zn, Fe, Cu and Mn) contents of various raw pig edible offal tissues (tongue, heart, lungs, liver, spleen, kidney, brain and spinal cord) are shown in Table 6. Overall, there are large variations in the mineral contents. Potassium is the highest for spleen (383.4-463.8 mg/100g), followed by spinal cord (317.1-377.4 mg/100g), brain and liver (253.2-387.8 mg/100g and 217-370.0 mg/100g, respectively), heart (175.7-300 mg/100g), tongue (243-258 mg/100g), lungs (222.5-303 mg/100g) and kidney (189-290 mg/100g). With the exception of spinal cord, with phosphorus content of somewhat higher than 500 mg/kg (501.4-502.0 mg/100g), the phosphorus content is highest in liver, where it ranges from 288 to 430.0 mg/100g. Brain is next highest in phosphorus content (282-363 mg/100g), followed by spleen (205-313.3 mg/100g), kidney (204-296.8 mg/100g), lungs (196-252.7 mg/100g), heart (160-245 mg/100g) and tongue (173.0-209.3 mg/100g).

Furthermore, lungs (144.1-163 mg/100g) and kidney (121-190 mg/100g) are the highest in sodium content. The content of sodium in spinal cord ranges from 125.8 to 146.0 mg/100g, while in brain it ranges from 120 to 158 mg/100g. Sodium is lowest in spleen (83.0-130 mg/100g), tongue (87.7-110 mg/100g), liver (71.6-150.0 mg/100g) and heart (56-110.8 mg/100g). All of the edible offal shown in Table 6 are consistently higher in sodium than pork meat (Table 4 and Table 5). Contents of magnesium are

Table 6. Mineral contents (mg/100g) of raw pig edible offal

Source	Edible offal	K	P	Na	Mg	Ca	Zn	Fe	Cu	Mn
Denmark – Danish Food Composition Database (2018)*	Tongue	282	195	92.0	18.0	6.52	2.60	2.15	0.230	0.034
	Heart	298	204	107	21.0	5.29	2.10	6.00	0.410	0.038
	Liver	271	369	80	18.0	6.48	6.78	13.4	1.01	0.390
	Kidney	244	238	160	18.0	6.97	2.59	3.30	0.715	0.150
Finland – Fineli - Finnish Food Composition Database (2018)*	Liver	370.0	430.0	150.0	24.0	6.0	9.0	31.4	–	–
	Kidney	230.0	260.0	165.0	18.0	9.0	2.3	8.4	–	–
Italy – Food Composition Database for Epidemiological Studies in Italy (2015)	Heart	300	245	80	25	35	2.30	5.3	0.47	0.03
	Liver	356	362	108	21	10	6.30	18.0	2.60	0.29
Lawrie and Ledward (2006)*	Liver	320	370	87	21	6	6.9	21.0	2.7	–
	Kidney	290	270	190	19	8	2.6	5.0	0.8	–
	Brain	270	340	140	15	12	1.2	1.6	0.3	–
Norway – The Norwegian Food Composition Table (2018)*	Heart	240	160	95	17	6	1.3	5.4	0.31	–
	Liver	287	411	94	20	5	8.7	18.04	0.64	–
USA – USDA Food Composition Databases (2018)*	Tongue	243	193	110	18	16	3.01	3.35	–	–
	Heart	294	169	56	19	5	2.8	4.68	–	–
	Lungs	303	196	153	14	7	2.03	18.90	–	–
	Liver	273	288	87	18	9	5.76	23.30	–	–
	Spleen	396	260	98	13	10	2.54	22.32	–	–
	Kidney	229	204	121	17	9	2.75	4.89	–	–
	Brain	258	282	120	14	10	1.27	1.60	–	–
Slovak Republic – Slovak Food Composition Database (2018)*	Tongue	258	192	104	23	11	2.6	4.28	–	–
	Heart	287	184	104	19	17	2.04	4.7	0.62	–
	Lungs	242	221	163	17	5.8	0.7	9.1	0.1	–
	Liver	317	353	115	24	8	6.64	15.34	2.6	–
	Spleen	401	205	130	34	9	2.6	19.8	0.2	–
	Kidney	249	260	184	21	8.5	1.7	6.8	0.5	–
	Brain	318	363	158	20	14.1	1.6	3.4	0.4	–
Republic of Serbia – Tomović et al., (2011b, 2013b); average of 10 genotypes*	Liver	217	383	82.2	25.7	20.4	9.82	21.8	1.61	0.35
	Kidney	189	287	130	23.3	20.2	2.99	7.42	1.29	0.22
Republic of Serbia – Jokanović et al., (2014); Tomović et al., (2014c); average of 5 purebreds*	Liver	218	388	85.2	26.3	20.9	10.1	22.3	1.78	0.36
	Kidney	193	288	134	23.6	20.2	3.01	7.48	1.28	0.22

Table 6. (Continued)

Source	Edible offal	K	P	Na	Mg	Ca	Zn	Fe	Cu	Mn
Tomović et al., (2016e)** Swallow-Belly Mangalica pigs, up to 150 kg LW	Tongue	245.8	173.0	87.7	17.4	12.79	2.13	2.56	0.238	0.036
	Heart	285.2	171.4	93.0	20.0	8.55	1.61	4.48	0.320	0.035
	Lungs	222.5	208.7	158.4	13.8	20.84	2.09	6.37	0.118	0.033
	Liver	359.0	344.5	80.2	20.4	13.59	5.34	33.58	0.365	0.267
	Spleen	463.8	301.4	83.0	18.0	5.36	3.15	27.49	0.205	0.045
	Kidney	247.7	225.8	157.2	19.1	13.02	2.24	5.96	0.393	0.123
	Brain	387.8	354.2	142.3	10.0	18.74	1.56	3.82	0.319	0.048
	Spinal cord	377.4	501.4	146.0	8.3	26.02	0.67	1.78	0.206	0.045
Tomović et al., (2016c)** Black Slavonian pigs, up to 130 kg LW	Heart	248	186	82.5	24.7	8.00	2.35	6.81	0.373	0.043
	Liver	301	315	71.6	28.5	7.84	6.47	45.59	0.379	0.254
	Kidney	266	256	127.7	25.5	9.61	3.16	9.33	0.362	0.152
Despotović et al., (2018a)** Swallow-Belly Mangalica pigs, up to 100 kg LW	Tongue	256.9	209.3	91.8	18.1	10.32	2.41	2.98	0.264	0.035
	Heart	175.7	232.3	110.8	21.8	8.32	2.83	5.10	0.391	0.039
	Lungs	225.6	252.7	144.1	14.0	12.99	1.95	8.81	0.154	0.032
	Liver	277.4	406.5	75.1	20.5	5.89	6.36	20.24	0.825	0.338
	Spleen	383.4	313.3	94.5	20.7	6.07	3.32	23.43	0.141	0.052
	Kidney	261.4	296.8	152.8	17.7	11.17	3.74	6.24	0.633	0.214
	Brain	253.2	359.9	123.3	15.0	7.60	3.97	2.51	0.440	0.050
	Spinal cord	317.1	502.0	125.8	14.2	17.21	0.79	2.30	0.257	0.060

* data for the commercial pigs; ** data for the indigenous pigs; LW – live weight.

similar for liver (18-28.5 mg/100g), spleen (13-34 mg/100g), heart (17-25 mg/100g), kidney (17-25.5 mg/100g) and tongue (17.4-23 mg/100g). The content of magnesium in brain and lungs ranges from 10.0 to 20 mg/100g and from 13.8 to 17 mg/100g, respectively. Spinal cord is the lowest in magnesium content (8.3-14.2 mg/100g). For given raw pig edible offal, spinal cord is markedly the highest in calcium content (17.21-26.02 mg/100g). Other raw edible offal (brain: 7.60-18.74 mg/100g; lungs: 5.8-20.84 mg/100g; heart: 5-35 mg/100g; kidney: 6.97-20.2 mg/100g; tongue: 6.52-16 mg/100g; liver: 5-20.9 mg/100g; spleen: 5.36-10 mg/100g) do not differ markedly in calcium content. There is, however, a wide variation in the calcium content for each type of raw pig edible offal. Liver and spleen are the best sources of iron. Values range from 13.4 to 45.59 mg/100g for liver and from 19.8 to 27.49 mg/100g for spleen. Also, lungs are the rich source of iron, with a content ranging from 6.37 to 18.90 mg/100g. Iron values are similar for kidney (3.30-9.33 mg/100g) and heart (4.48-6.81 mg/100g), and for tongue (2.15-4.28 mg/100g) and brain (1.60-3.82 mg/100g). The lowest amount of iron is for spinal cord (1.78-2.30 mg/100g). All of the pig edible offal shown in Table 6 have iron content greater or equal to that for pork meat (Table 4 and Table 5). Liver is the richest source of zinc, and values range from 5.34 to 10.1 mg/100g. These values are on average three times higher than amount in pork meat (Table 4 and Table 5). Values for spleen, kidney, tongue, heart, brain and lungs are in the ranges: 2.54-3.32 mg/100g, 1.7-3.74 mg/100g, 2.13-3.01 mg/100g, 1.3-2.83 mg/100g, 1.2-3.97 mg/100g and 0.7-2.09 mg/100g, respectively. Spinal cord is the lowest in zinc content (0.67-0.79 mg/100g). Copper is the highest for liver (0.365-2.7 mg/100g). Otherwise, it is in the range: 0.362-1.29 mg/100g (kidney), 0.31-0.62 mg/100g (heart), 0.3-0.440 mg/100g (brain), 0.230-0.264 mg/100g (tongue), 0.206-0.257 mg/100g (spinal cord), 0.141–0.205 mg/100g (spleen) and 0.1–0.154 mg/100g (lungs). Liver and kidney contain markedly more copper than pork meat (Table 4 and Table 5). Of the raw pig edible offal with values for manganese, liver and kidney contain the highest amounts. Content ranges from 0.254 to 0.390 mg/100g in liver and from 0.123 to 0.22 mg/100g in kidney. The remaining raw pig edible offal contain less than 0.1 mg/100g manganese. Manganese levels in spinal cord, brain,

Table 7. Mineral contents (mg/100g) of raw pig fatty tissue

Source	Fatty tissue	K	P	Na	Ca	Mg	Zn	Fe	Cu	Mn
US – USDA Food	Lard	0.02	–	0.01	0.07	0.02	0.11	–	–	–
Composition Databases (2018)*	Leaf fat	31	19	5	1	1	0.18	0.09	–	–
Hopkins and Murphy (1962)*	Fat (pork leg)	–	–	18.0	2.2	–	–	0.3	0.02	–
Honikel (2011)*	Lard	1	3	2	1	1	0.1	0.05	0.02	–
Tomović et al., (2014b)** Swallow-Belly Mangalica	Lard (back fat)	15.58	17.74	8.83	3.36	1.08	0.32	0.42	0.06	0.007
pigs, up to 150 kg LW	Leaf fat	16.20	17.02	8.65	3.29	1.23	0.39	0.53	0.05	0.009

* data for the commercial pigs; ** data for the indigenous pigs; LW – live weight.

spleen, heart, tongue and lungs range from 0.03 mg/100g (heart) to 0.06 mg/100g (spinal cord). For a number of items listed, no values for manganese were available. The manganese content of the liver and kidney are markedly higher than those of pork meat (Table 4 and Table 5).

Corresponding data for the mineral (K, P, Na, Mg, Ca, Zn, Fe, Cu and Mn) contents of various raw fatty tissues (lard and leaf fat) are shown in Table 7. Compared to pork meat (Table 4 and Table 5) and pig edible offal (Table 6), the mineral contents of fatty tissues is markedly lower.

COOKED PORK MEAT

Meat is commonly cooked prior to consumption. Cooking can be described as the practice of preparing food for eating by the application of heat (Carmody and Wrangham, 2009). The method of cooking is one of the major factors that affect the eating quality of meat. Meat is cooked using different media for heat transfer, such as dry heat methods (roasting, broiling or pan-frying), moist heating methods (boiling or braising) or microwave cooking (electromagnetic energy) (Bejerholm and Aaslyng, 2004). The selection of the cooking treatment must take into account the meat type, the amount of connective tissue, and the shape and size of meat. Despite cooking treatment, cooking temperature is one of the well-known altering factors that can influence the characteristics of meat products. The temperature on the surface of meat, the temperature profile through the meat, and the method of heat transfer are the most important differences across the cooking methods (Alfaia et al., 2013; Bejerholm and Aaslyng, 2004).

Meat composition, as well as its physico-chemical properties, undergoes significant changes during heat treatment. It is well known that cooking time, temperature and cooking method have a great effect on eating quality indicators including tenderness, juiciness, flavour, colour and overall acceptability of pork meat (Heymann et al., 1990; Wood et al., 1995; Aaslyng et al., 2003; Tornberg, 2005; Christensen et al., 2011; Huang et al., 2011; Alfaia et al., 2013). Moreover cooking is a critical process to assure microbiological and chemical safety of meat products (Tornberg, 2005; Alfaia et al., 2013).

Number of authors (Rhee et al., 1993; Lombardi-Boccia et al., 2005; Gerber et al., 2009; Greenfield et al., 2009; van Heerden and Smith, 2013; Tomović et al., 2015a, 2016d) pointed out that the cooking process can affect the mineral composition of pork meat in various ways and to different degrees by changing the nutritional value of cooked products in relation to raw samples. According to Rhee et al., (1993), overall retention of minerals in cooked meat varied from 84 to 96%. van Heerden and Smith (2013) did not obtain significant differences in mineral contents between raw and cooked pork meat, except for zinc. Results obtained by Gerber et al., (2009), calculated in absolute terms based on an initial 100 g of raw pork meat, show that contents of phosphorus, potassium, sodium, magnesium, calcium and zinc decreased during cooking, while iron content was reported to increase. Investigating the effect of endpoint internal temperature (51, 61, 71, 81 and 91°C) on mineral contents of boiled pork loin Tomović et al., (2015a) concluded that: all boiling treatments led to significantly increased mineral contents, except for potassium and sodium, compared to raw meat; as endpoint temperature was increased, mineral contents increased, reaching numerically or significantly highest contents at: 61°C for sodium and magnesium, 71°C for phosphorus, potassium, calcium, zinc, copper and manganese, and 81°C for iron, after which mineral contents decreased. In addition, investigating the effect of endpoint internal temperature (51, 61, 71, 81 and 91°C) on mineral contents of roasted pork loin Tomović et al., (2016d) concluded that: all roasting treatments led to significantly increased mineral contents, except for sodium, compared to raw meat; as endpoint temperature was increased, mineral contents increased, reaching numerically or significantly highest contents at 61°C for calcium, 71°C for manganese and 91°C for phosphorous, potassium, sodium, magnesium, zinc, iron and copper. The values for mineral content in roasted pork loin obtained by Tomović et al., (2015a) are in agreement with the results reported by Greenfield et al., (2009). Similar trend in mineral content was also obtained by Lombardi-Boccia et al., (2005), who investigated the effects of cooking on zinc, iron and copper contents in pork meat.

20 *Vladimir Tomović, Mila Tomović, Branislav Šojić et al.*

Published information on mineral retention during cooking in pig edible offal is scant. Mineral retention for pig edible offal may not always be similar to those of pork meat. Potassium and sodium tend to decrease, phosphorous, magnesium, iron and manganese are not consistent in their direction of change, while zinc content increase during cooking of pig edible offal (Anderson, 1988).

ACKNOWLEDGMENTS

This work was supported by the Ministry of Education, Science and Technological Development of Republic of Serbia, project TR31032.

REFERENCES

Aaslyng, M. D., Bejerholm, C., Ertbjerg, P., Bertram, H. C. and Andersen, H. J. (2003). Cooking loss and juiciness of pork in relation to raw meat quality and cooking procedure. *Food Quality and Preference*, 14 (4): 277-88.

Alfaia, C. M., Lopes, A. F., and Prates, J. A. M. 2013. "Cooking and Diet Quality: A Focus on Meat." In *Diet Quality, an Evidence-Based Approach*, edited by Victor R. Preedy, Lan-Anh Hunter, and Vinood B. Patel, 257-84, New York: Humana Press. (Alfaia, Lopes and Prates 2013, 257-84).

Anderson, B. A. 1988. "Composition and Nutritional Value of Edible Meat By-Products." In *Edible Meat By-Products, Advances in Meat Research*, edited by Albert M. Pearson, and Thayne R. Dutson, Vol. 5, 15-45. London: Elsevier Science Publishers Ltd. (Anderson 1988, 15-45).

Bejerholm, C., and Aaslyng, M. D. 2004. "Cooking of Meat." In *Encyclopedia of Meat Sciences*, edited by Werner K. Jensen, Carrick Devine, and Michael Dikeman, 343-9, Oxford: Elsevier Science Ltd. (Bejerholm and Aaslyng 2004, 343-9).

Macro- and Micromineral Contents in Raw ...

Belitz, Hans-Dieter, Werner Grosch, and Peter Schieberle. 2009. *Food Chemistry (4th revised and extended ed.)*. Berlin and Heidelberg: Springer-Verlag. (Belitz, Grosch and Schieberle 2009, 421-8).

Carmody, R. N. and Wrangham, R. W. (2009). The energetic significance of cooking. *Journal of Human Evolution*, 57 (4): 379-91.

Christensen, L., Ertbjerg, P., Aaslyng, M. D. and Christensen, M. (2011). Effect of prolonged heat treatment from 48°C to 63°C on toughness, cooking loss and color of pork. *Meat Science*, 88 (2): 280-5.

Dabrowski, W. M. 2004. "Introduction." In *Toxins in Food*, edited by Waldemar M. Dabrowski, and Zdzislaw E. Sikorski, 1-10. Boca Raton, London, New York, Washington, D.C.: CRC Press. (Dabrowski 2004, 1-10).

Dabrowski, Waldemar M., and Zdzislaw E. Sikorski. 2004. *Toxins in Food*. Boca Raton, London, New York, Washington, D.C.: CRC Press. (Dabrowski and Zdzislaw 2004).

Danish Food Composition Database. 2018. Accessed October 18. https://frida.fooddata.dk/?lang=en.

Davies, A. S. 2004. "Muscle Structure and Contraction." In *Encyclopedia of Meat Sciences*, edited by Werner K. Jensen, Carrick Devine, and Michael Dikeman, 882-901. Oxford: Elsevier Science Ltd. (Davies 2004, 882-901).

Despotović, A., Tomović, V., Šević, R., Jokanović, M., Stanišić, N., Škaljac, S., Šojić, B., Hromiš, N, Stajić, S. and Petrović, J. (2018b). Meat quality traits of *M. longissimus lumborum* from White Mangalica and (Duroc x White Mangalica) x White Mangalica pigs reared under intensive conditions and slaughtered at about 180-kg live weight. *Italian Journal of Animal Science*, in press, DOI: 10.1080/1828051X.2018.1443287.

Despotović, A., Tomović, V., Stanišić, N., Jokanović, M., Šojić, B., Škaljac, S., Tomašević, I., Stajić, S., Martinović, A. and Hromiš, N. (2018a). Edible offal quality of Swallow-Belly Mangalica pigs reared under an intensive production system – investigation on pigs slaughtered at 100 kg live weight. *Fleischwirtschaft International*, 5: 49-54.

FAOSTAT. 2018. *The Food and Agriculture Organization of the United Nations*. Accessed October 18. www.fao.org/faostat/en/#home.

Fineli - Finnish Food Composition Database. 2018. Accessed October 18. https://fineli.fi/fineli/en/index.

Food Composition Database for Epidemiological Studies in Italy. 2015. Accessed October 18. http://www.bda-ieo.it/wordpress/en/.

Galián, M., Peinado, B., Martínez, C., Periago, M. J., Ros, G. and Poto, A. (2007). Comparative study of the characteristics of the carcass and the meat of the Chato Murciano pig and its cross with Iberian pig, reared indoors. *Animal Science Journal*, 78 (6): 659-67.

Galián, M., Poto, A. and Peinado, B. (2009). Carcass and meat quality traits of the Chato Murciano pig slaughtered at different weights. *Livestock Science*, 124 (1-3): 314-20.

Gerber, N., Scheeder, M. R. L. and Wenk, C. (2009). The influence of cooking and fat trimming on the actual nutrient intake from meat. *Meat Science*, 81 (1): 148-54.

Greaser, M. L. 2001. "Postmortem Muscle Chemistry." In *Meat Science and Applications*, edited by Yiu H. Hui, Wai-Kit Nip, Robert W. Rogers, and Owen A. Young, 21-37. New York, Basel: Marcel Dekker, Inc. (Greaser 2001, 21-37).

Greenfield, H., Arcot, J., Barnes, J. A., Cunningham, J., Adorno, P., Stobaus, T., Tume, R. K., Beilken, S. L. and Muller, W. J. (2009). Nutrient composition of Australian retail pork cuts 2005/2006. *Food Chemistry*, 117 (4): 721-30.

Greenfield, Heather, and David A. T. Southgate. (2003). *Food composition data: Production, management and use (2nd ed.).* Rome: Food and Agriculture Organisation of the United Nations. (Greenfield and Southgate 2003, 63-82, 187-97).

Hermida, M., Gonzalez, M., Miranda, M. and Rodríguez-Otero, J. L. (2006). Mineral analysis in rabbit meat from Galicia (NW Spain). *Meat Science*, 73 (4): 635-9.

Heymann, H., Hendrick, H. B., Karrasch, M. A., Eggeman, M. K. and Ellersieck, M. R. (1990). Sensory and chemical characteristics of fresh pork roasts cooked to different endpoint temperatures. *Journal of Food Science*, 55 (3): 613-7.

Honikel, K. O. (1999). Biochemical and physico-chemical characteristics of meat quality. *Tehnologija mesa*, 40 (3-5): 105-23.

Honikel, K. O. (2011). "Composition and Calories." In *Handbook of Analysis of Edible Animal By-Products*, edited by Leo M. L. Nollet, and Fidel Toldrá, 105-21. Boca Raton, London, New York: CRC Press, Taylor and Francis Group. (Honikel 2011, 105-21).

Hopkins, H. T. and Murphy, E. W. (1962). Mineral content of meats, mineral elements in adipose tissue of lamb and pork. *Journal of Agricultural and Food Chemistry*, 10 (6): 515-7.

Huang, F., Huang, M., Xu, X. and Zhou, G. (2011). Influence of heat on protein degradation, ultrastructure and eating quality indicators of pork. *Journal of the Science of Food and Agriculture*, 91 (3): 443-8.

Jensen, W.K., Devine, C., and Dikeman, M. 2004. "Introduction." In *Encyclopedia of Meat Sciences*, edited by Werner K. Jensen, Carrick Devine, and Michael Dikeman, xi-xii. Oxford: Elsevier Science Ltd. (Jensen, Devine and Dikeman 2004, xi-xii).

Jokanović, M. R., Tomović, V. M., Šojić, B. V., Škaljac, S. B., Tasić, T. A., Ikonić, P. M. and Kevrešan, Ž. S. (2013). Cadmium in meat and edible offal of free-range reared Swallow-Belly Mangulica pigs from Vojvodina (northern Serbia). *Food Additives and Contaminants Part B: Surveillance*, 6 (2): 98-102.

Jokanović, Marija, Vladimir Tomović, Žarko Kevrešan, Mila Tomović, Snežana Škaljac, Branislav Šojić, Tatjana Tasić, Predrag Ikonić, Nevena Hromiš, and Aleksandra Martinović. 2014. "Content of macro elements in the liver and kidney from five modern purebred pigs produced in Vojvodina (northern Serbia)." Paper presented at *the 7th Central European Congress on Food "Food Chain Integration," 68-9, Ohrid, Macedonia, May 21-24*.

Lawrie, Ralston A., and David A. Ledward. 2006. *Lawrie's meat science (7th ed.)*. Cambridge: Woodhead Publishing Ltd. and CRC Press LLC. (Lawrie and Ledward 2004, 1-14, 75-127).

Leth, T. 2004. "Major Meat Components." In *Encyclopedia of Meat Sciences*, edited by Werner K. Jensen, Carrick Devine, and Michael Dikeman, 185-90. Oxford: Elsevier Science Ltd. (Leth 2004, 185-90).

24 *Vladimir Tomović, Mila Tomović, Branislav Šojić et al.*

Lombardi-Boccia, G., Lanzi, S. and Aguzzi, A. (2005). Aspects of meat quality: trace elements and B vitamins in raw and cooked meats. *Journal of Food Composition and Analysis*, 18 (1): 39-46.

Nollet, L. M., and Toldrá, F. 2011. Introduction – Offal Meat: Definitions, Regions, Cultures, and Generalities. In *Handbook of Analysis of Edible Animal By-Products*, edited by Leo M. L. Nollet, and Fidel Toldrá, 3-11. Boca Raton, London, New York: CRC Press, Taylor and Francis Group. (Nollet and Toldrá 2011, 3-11).

Ockerman, H. W., and Basu, L. 2004. "Edible, for Human Consumption." In *Encyclopedia of Meat Sciences*, edited by Werner K. Jensen, Carrick Devine, and Michael Dikeman, 104-12. Oxford: Elsevier Science Ltd. (Ockerman and Basu 2004, 104-12).

Ognjanović, Aleksandar, Sonja Karan-Đurić, Radomir Radovanović, and Vladimir Perić. 1985. *Tehnologija pratećih proizvoda industrije mesa*. Beograd: Univerzitet u Beogradu, Poljoprivredni fakultet. [*Technology of the by-products from the meat industry*. Belgrade: University of Belgrade, Faculty of Agriculture]. (Ognjanović, Karan-Đurić, Radovanović and Perić 1985, 103-139).

Olsson, V. and Pickova, J. (2005). The influence of production systems on meat quality, with emphasis on pork. *Ambio*, 34 (4-5): 338-43.

Poto, A., Galián, M. and Peinado, B. (2007). Chato Murciano pig and its crosses with Iberian and Large White pigs, reared outdoors. Comparative study of the carcass and meat characteristics. *Livestock Science*, 111 (1-2): 96-103.

Reilly, C. 2002. "Minerals." In *The Nutrition Handbook for Food Processors*, edited by Christiani Jeyakumar K. Henry, and Clare Chapman, 97-116. Boca Raton, Boston, New York, Washington, D.C., Cambridge: CRC Press and Woodhead Publishing Ltd. (Reilly 2002, 97-116).

Rhee, K. S., Griffith-Bradle, H. A. and Ziprin, Y. A. (1993). Nutrient composition and retention in browned ground beef, lamb, and pork. *Journal of Food Composition and Analysis*, 6 (3): 268-77.

Rosenvold, K. and Andersen, H. J. (2003). Factors of significance for pork quality – a review. *Meat Science*, 64 (3): 219-37.

Serbian Regulation. 1985. Pravilnik o kvalitetu zaklanih svinja i kategorizaciji svinjskog mesa. *Službeni list SFRJ*, 2: 20-30. [Rules on quality of slaughtered pigs and categorization of pig meat. *Official Gazette of the SFRY*, 2: 20-30].

Slovak Food Composition Database. 2018. Accessed October 18. http://www.pbd-online.sk/en.

Smith, S. B., Smith, D. R., and Lunt, D. K. 2004. "Adipose Tissue." In *Encyclopedia of Meat Sciences*, edited by Werner K. Jensen, Carrick Devine, and Michael Dikeman, 225-38. Oxford: Elsevier Science Ltd. (Smith, Smith and Lunt 2004, 225-38).

Spooncer, W. F. 1988. "Organs and Glands as Human Food." In *Edible Meat By-Products, Advances in Meat Research*, edited by Albert M. Pearson, and Thayne R. Dutson, Vol. 5, 197-217. London: Elsevier Science Publishers Ltd. (Spooncer 1988, 197-217).

Swartz, D. R., Greaser, M. L., and Cantino, M. E. 2009. "Muscle Structure and Function." In *Applied Muscle Biology and Meat Science*, edited by Min Du, and Richard J. McCormick, 1-45. Boca Raton: CRC Press, Taylor and Francis Group. (Swartz, Greaser, and Cantino 2009, 1-45).

The National Academy of Sciences, The Health and Medicine Division, USA, 2018. *Dietary Reference Intakes Tables and Application.* Accessed October 18. http://nationalacademies.org/hmd/Activities/Nutrition/SummaryDRIs/DRI-Tables.aspx.

The Norwegian Food Composition Tables, 2018. Accessed October 18. http://www.matportalen.no/verktoy/the_norwegian_food_composition_table/.

Toldrá, F., Aristoy, M. -C., Mora, L. and Reig, M. (2012). Innovations in value-addition of edible meat by-products. *Meat Science*, 92 (3): 290-6.

Tomović, V. M, Petrović, Lj. S., Tomović, M. S., Kevrešan, Ž. S., Jokanović, M. R., Džinić, N. R. and Despotović, A. R. (2011a). Cadmium concentration in the liver of 10 different pig genetic lines from Vojvodina, Serbia. *Food Additives and Contaminants Part B: Surveillance*, 4 (3): 180-4.

Tomović, V. M., Jokanović, M. R., Tomović, M. S., Šojić, B. V., Škaljac, S. B., Tasić, T. A., and Ikonić, P. M. 2013a. "Cadmium Level in Red Meat and Edible Offal." In *Cadmium: Characteristics, Sources of Exposure, Health and Environmental Effects*, edited by M Hasanuzzaman, and M Fujita, 341-8. New York: Nova Publishers. (Tomović, Jokanović, Tomović, Šojić, Škaljac, Tasić and Ikonić 2013, 341-8)

Tomović, V. M., Petrović, Lj. S., Tomović, M. S., Kevrešan, Ž. S. and Džinić, N. R. (2011b): Determination of mineral contents of semimembranosus muscle and liver from pure and crossbred pigs in Vojvodina (northern Serbia). *Food Chemistry*, 124 (1): 342-8.

Tomović, V. M., Petrović, Lj. S., Tomović, M. S., Kevrešan, Ž. S., Jokanović, M. R., Džinić, N. R. and Despotović, A. R. (2011c). Cadmium levels of kidney from 10 different pig genetic lines in Vojvodina (northern Serbia). *Food Chemistry*, 129 (1): 100-3.

Tomović, V. M., Šević, R., Jokanović, M., Šojić, B., Škaljac, S., Tasić, T., Ikonić, P., Lušnic Polak, M., Polak, T. and Demšar, L. (2016b). Quality traits of *longissimus lumborum* muscle from White Mangalica, Duroc x White Mangalica and Large White pigs reared under intensive conditions and slaughtered at 150 kg live weight: a comparative study. *Archives Animal Breeding*, 59: 401-15.

Tomović, V. M., Stanišić, N. Z., Jokanović, M. R., Kevrešan, Ž. S., Šojić, B. V., Škaljac, S. B., Tomašević, I. B., Martinović, A. B., Despotović, A. R. and Šuput, D. Z. (2016a). Meat quality of Swallow-Belly Mangulica pigs reared under intensive production system and slaughtered at 100 kg live weight. *Hemijska Industrija*, 70 (5): 557-64.

Tomović, V. M., Vujadinović, D. D., Grujić, R. P., Jokanović, M. R., Kevrešan, Ž. S., Škaljac, S. B., Šojić, B. V., Tasić, T. A., Ikonić, P. M. and Hromiš, N. M. (2015a). Effect of endpoint internal temperature on mineral contents of boiled pork loin. *Journal of Food Processing and Preservation*, 39 (6): 1854-8.

Tomović, V. M., Žlender, B. A., Jokanović, M. R., Tomović, M. M., Šojić, B. V., Škaljac, S. B., Kevrešan, Ž. S., Tasić, T. A., Ikonić, P. M. and Šošo, M. M. (2014a). Sensory, physical and chemical characteristics of meat from free-range reared Swallow-belly Mangulica pigs. *Journal of Animal and Plant Sciences*, 24 (3): 704-13.

Tomović, V., Jokanović, M., Kevrešan, Ž., Škaljac, S., Šojić, B., Tasić, T., Ikonić, P., Živković, D., Stajić, S. and Hromiš, N. (2015b). Content of macrominerals in the *M. semimembranosus* and *M. longissimus thoracis et lumborum* from five purebred pigs produced in Vojvodina. *Journal on Processing and Energy in Agriculture*, 19 (2): 87-90.

Tomović, V., Jokanović, M., Kevrešan, Ž., Škaljac, S., Šojić, B., Tasić, T., Ikonić, P., Škrinjar, M., Lazić, V. and Tomović, M. (2014b). Physical characteristics and proximate and mineral composition of adipose tissue from free-range reared Swallow-Belly Mangulica pigs from Vojvodina. *Journal on Processing and Energy in Agriculture*, 18 (4): 187-90.

Tomović, V., Mastanjević, K., Kovačević, D., Jokanović, M., Kevrešan, Ž., Škaljac, S., Šojić, B., Lukač, D., Škrobot, D. and Despotović, A. (2016c). Proximate and mineral composition and cadmium content of main anatomical parts and offal from semi-outdoor reared Black Slavonian pigs. *Agro FOOD Industry Hi Tech*, 27 (6): 39-42.

Tomović, V., Petrović, Lj., Jokanović, M., Tomović, M., Kevrešan, Ž., Tasić, T., Ikonić, P., Šojić, B., Škaljac, S. and Šošo, M. (2013b). Mineral concentration of the kidney in ten different pig genetic lines from Vojvodina (northern Serbia). *Acta Alimentaria*, 42 (2): 198-207.

Tomović, V., Vujadinović, D., Grujić, R., Jokanović, M., Kevrešan, Ž., Škaljac, S., Šojić, B., Vasilev, D., Kocić-Tanackov, S. and Hromiš, N. (2016d). Effect of endpoint internal temperature on mineral contents of roasted pork loin. *Fleischwirtschaft International*, 6: 101-5.

Tomović, V., Žlender, B., Jokanović, M., Tomović, M., Šojić, B., Škaljac, S., Kevrešan, Ž., Tasić, T., Ikonić, P. and Okanović, Đ. (2016e). Physical and chemical characteristics of edible offal from free-range reared Swallow-Belly Mangalica pigs. *Acta Alimentaria*, 45 (2): 190-7.

Tomović, Vladimir, Marija Jokanović, Žarko Kevrešan, Branislav Šojić, Snežana Škaljac, Tatjana Tasić, Predrag Ikonić, Dušan Živković, Slaviša Stajić, and Ivana Lončarević. 2015c. "Content of microminerals in the *M. semimembranosus* and *M. longissimus thoracis et lumborum* from pigs produced in Vojvodina." Paper presented at the *IV International Congress "Engineering, Ecology and Materials in the*

Processing Industry," *432-7, Jahorina, Bosnia and Herzegovina, March 04- 06.*

Tomović, Vladimir, Marija Jokanović, Žarko Kevrešan, Mila Tomović, Snežana Škaljac, Branislav Šojić, Tatjana Tasić, Predrag Ikonić, Nevena Hromiš, and Aleksandra Martinović. 2014c. "Content of micro elements in the liver and kidney from five modern purebred pigs produced in Vojvodina (northern Serbia)." Paper presented at the *7th Central European Congress on Food "Food Chain Integration," 90, Ohrid, Macedonia, May 21-24.*

Tornberg, E. (2005). Effects of heat on meat proteins – Implications on structure and quality of meat products. *Meat Science*, 70 (3): 493-508.

U.S. FDA. 2000. U.S. Food and Drug Administration. Accessed October 18. https://www.fda.gov/default.htm.

USDA - Food Composition Databases. 2018. Accessed October 18. https://ndb.nal.usda.gov/ndb/search/list?home=true.

van Heerden, S. M. and Smith, M. F. (2013). The nutrient composition of three cuts obtained from P-class South African pork carcasses. *Food Chemistry*, 140 (3): 458-65.

Williamson, C. S., Foster, R. K., Stanner, S. A. and Buttriss, J. L. (2005). Red meat in the diet. *Nutrition Bulletin*, 30 (4): 323-55.

Wood, J. D., Enser, M., Fisher, A. V., Nute, G. R., Sheard, P. R., Richardson, R. I., Hughes, S. I. and Whittington, F. M. (2008). Fat deposition, fatty acid composition and meat quality: A review. *Meat Science*, 78 (4): 343-58.

Wood, J. D., Nute, G. R., Fursey, G. A. J. and Cuthbertson, A. (1995). The effect of cooking conditions on the eating quality of pork. *Meat Science*, 40 (2): 127-35.

BIOGRAPHICAL SKETCH

Vladimir Tomović, PhD

Affiliation: University of Novi Sad, Faculty of Technology Novi Sad, Department of Food Preservation Engineering, Novi Sad, Serbia

Education:

BSc – 2000, University of Novi Sad, Faculty of Technology Novi Sad, Serbia

MSc – 2002, University of Novi Sad, Faculty of Technology Novi Sad, Serbia

PhD – 2009, University of Novi Sad, Faculty of Technology Novi Sad, Serbia

Research and Professional Experience:

Associate Professor, Vladimir Tomović, is scientist in the field of meat production and processing, food preservation, sensory evaluation of food, and nutritional value of food. In his scientific work he specially deals with pig carcass quality evaluation, as well as, with influences of different premortal and postmortal factors on meat and carcass quality. Furthermore, he studies technological, nutritional, sensory, hygienic and toxicological aspects of meat quality (pork, beef and poultry). Also, his research is focused on development of chilling, curing, salting and drying technology of meat products, all with the same final aim – safety of meat and meat products. He pays special attention to the valorization of meat industry edible byproducts (offal) as potential sources of nutritional elements in human diet, and development of equipment and new technologies in meat production and processing. He was leader or participant in number of international (8) and national (12) projects. He teaches at undergraduate (BSc) and postgraduate (MSc and PhD) levels, and was mentor of 20 undergraduates and 9 postgraduates (6 MSc and 3 PhD). He is the author of more than 350 published scientific papers, one monograph, two book chapters, one workbook exercise and one classbook.

Professional Appointments:

Senior Technical Associate – 2000-2001, University of Novi Sad, Faculty of Technology Novi Sad, Serbia

Assistant Trainee – 2001-2004, University of Novi Sad, Faculty of Technology Novi Sad, Serbia

30 *Vladimir Tomović, Mila Tomović, Branislav Šojić et al.*

Assistant – 2004-2010, University of Novi Sad, Faculty of Technology Novi
Sad, Serbia
Assistant Professor – 2010-2015, University of Novi Sad, Faculty of
Technology Novi Sad, Serbia
Associate Professor – 2015-Current, University of Novi Sad, Faculty of
Technology Novi Sad, Serbia

Honors: Special Award of the Serbian Chemical Society for 2000 year

Publications from the Last 3 Years:

Book Chapters
Petrović, Lj., Tasić, T., Ikonić, P., Šojić, B., Škaljac, S., Danilović, B.,
Jokanović, M., Tomović, V., and Džinić, N. (2016). Quality
Standardization of Traditional Dry Fermented Sausages: Case of
Petrovská klobása. In *Emerging and Traditional Technologies for Safe,
Healthy and Quality Food,* edited by Viktor Nedović, Peter Raspor,
Jovanka Lević, Vesna Tumbas Šaponjac, Gustavo V. Barbosa-Cánovas,
221-34, Springer International Publishing, Switzerland.

New Product or Technology or Technical Solutions
Vasilev, D., Jovetić, M., Korićanac, V., Tomović, V., Jokanović, M.,
Dimitrijević, M., and Vasiljević, N. (2016). *Funkcionalna fermentisana
kobasica sa smanjenim sadržajem natrijuma i povećanim sadržajem
kalijuma "Probio-K"* (*Functional fermented sausage with reduced
sodium content and enriched with potassium "Probio-K"*) (in Serbian).
Vasilev, D., Jovetić, M., Vranić, D., Tomović, V., Jokanović, M., Karabasil,
N., and Vasiljević, N. (2016). *Funkcionalna fermentisana kobasica sa
smanjenim sadržajem natrijuma i povećanim sadržajem kalcijuma i
kalijuma "Probio-Ca"* (*Functional fermented sausage with reduced
sodium content and enriched with calcium and potassium "Probio-Ca"*)
(in Serbian).

Published Papers – In the Leading International Journals

Despotović, A., Tomović, V., Šević, R., Jokanović, M., Stanišić, N., Škaljac, S., Šojić, B., Hromiš, N., Stajić, S. and Petrović, J. (2018). Meat quality traits of M. longissimus lumborum from White Mangalica and (Duroc x White Mangalica) x White Mangalica pigs reared under intensive conditions and slaughtered at about 180-kg live weight. *Italian Journal of Animal Science*, in press: DOI: 10.1080/1828051X.2018.1443287.

Hromiš, N., Lazić, V., Popović, S., Markov, S., Vaštag, Ž., Šuput, D., Bulut, S. and Tomović, V. (2016). Investigation of a product-specific active packaging material based on chitosan biofilm with spice oleoresin. *Journal of Food and Nutrition Research*, 55 (1): 78-88.

Ikonić, P., Jokanović, M., Petrović, Lj., Tasić, T., Škaljac, S., Šojić, B., Džinić, N., Tomović, V., Tomić, J., Danilović, B. and Ikonić, B. (2016). Effect of starter culture addition and processing method on proteolysis and texture profile of traditional dry-fermented sausage Petrovská klobása. *International Journal of Food Properties*, 19 (9): 1924-37.

Kocić-Tanackov, S., Dimić, G., Mojović, Lj., Gvozdanović-Varga, J., Djukić-Vuković, A., Tomović, V., Šojić, B. and Pejin, J. (2017). Antifungal activity of the onion (*Allium cepa* L.) essential oil against Aspergillus, Fusarium and Penicillium species isolated from food. *Journal of Food Processing and Preservation*, 41 (4): e13050.

Nikolić, I., Dokić, Lj., Rakić, D., Tomović, V., Maravić, N., Vidosavljević, S., Šereš, Z. and Šoronja-Simović, D. (2018). The role of two types of continuous phases based on cellulose during textural, color and sensory characterization of novel food spread with pumpkin seed flour. *Journal of Food Processing and Preservation*, 42 (8): in press: DOI: 10.1111/jfpp.13684.

Polak, T., Lušnic Polak, M., Tomović, V., Žlender, B. and Demšar, L. (2017). Characterisation of the kranjska klobasa, a traditional slovenian cooked, cured, and smoked sausage from coarse ground pork. *Journal of Food Processing and Preservation*, 41 (6): e13269.

Škaljac, S., Jokanović, M., Tomović, V., Ivić, M., Tasić, T., Ikonić, P., Šojić, B., Džinić, N. and Petrović, Lj. (2018). Influence of smoking in traditional and industrial conditions on colour and content of polycyclic aromatic hydrocarbons in dry fermented sausage "*Petrovská klobása.*" *LWT - Food Science and Technology*, 87: 158-62.

Škaljac, S., Petrović, Lj., Jokanović, M., Tasić, T., Ivić, M., Tomović, V., Ikonić, P., Šojić, B., Džinić, N. and Škrbić, B. (2018). Influence of collagen and natural casings on the polycyclic aromatic hydrocarbons in traditional dry fermented sausage (*Petrovská klobása*) from Serbia. *International Journal of Food Properties*, 21 (1): 667-73.

Škunca, D., Tomašević, I., Nastasijević, I., Tomović, V. and Djekić, I. (2018). Life cycle assessment of the chicken meat chain. *Journal of Cleaner Production*, 184: 440-50.

Šojić, B., Pavlić, B., Zeković, Z., Tomović, V., Ikonić, P., Kocić-Tanackov, S. and Džinić, N. (2018). The effect of essential oil and extract from sage (*Salvia officinalis* L.) herbal dust (food industry by-product) on the oxidative and microbiological stability of fresh pork sausages. *LWT - Food Science and Technology*, 89: 749-55.

Šojić, B., Tomović, V., Kocić-Tanackov, S., Škaljac, S., Ikonić, P., Džinić, N., Živković, N., Jokanović, M., Tasić, T. and Kravić, S. (2015). Effect of nutmeg (*Myristica fragrans*) essential oil on the oxidative and microbial stability of cooked sausage during refrigerated storage. *Food Control*, 54: 282-6.

Stajić, S., Stanišić, N., Lević, S., Tomović, V., Lilić, S., Vranić, D., Jokanović, M. and Živković, D. (2018). Physico-chemical characteristics and sensory quality of dry fermented sausages with flaxseed oil preparations. *Polish Journal of Food and Nutrition Sciences*, 68 (4): 367-75.

Tomasević, I., Tomović, V., Milovanović, B., Lorenzo, J., Đorđević, V., Karabasil, N. Djekić, I. (2019). Comparison of a computer vision system vs. traditional colorimeter for color evaluation of meat products with various physical properties. *Meat Science*, 148, 5-12.

Tomović, V., Jokanović, M., Tomović, M., Lazović, M., Šojić, B., Škaljac, S., Ivić, M., Kocić-Tanackov, S., Tomašević, I. and Martinović, A. (2017). Cadmium and lead in female cattle livers and kidneys from Vojvodina, northern Serbia. *Food Additives and Contaminants Part B: Surveillance*, 10 (1): 39-43.

Tomović, V., Jokanović, M., Tomović, M., Lazović, M., Šojić, B., Škaljac, S., Ivić, M., Kocić-Tanackov, S., Tomašević, I. and Martinović, A. (2017). Cadmium in liver and kidneys of domestic Balkan and Alpine dairy goat breeds from Montenegro and Serbia. *Food Additives and Contaminants Part B: Surveillance*, 10 (2): 137-42.

Tomović, V. M., Jokanović, M. R., Švarc-Gajić, J. V., Vasiljević, I. M., Šojić, B. V., Škaljac, S. B., Pihler, I. I., Simin, V. B., Krajinović, M. M. and Žujović, M. M. (2016). Physical characteristics and proximate and mineral composition of Saanen goat male kids meat from Vojvodina (Northern Serbia) as influenced by muscle. *Small Ruminant Research*, 145: 44-52.

Published Papers – In International Journals

Despotović, A., Tomović, V., Stanišić, N., Jokanović, M., Šojić, B., Škaljac, S., Tomašević, I., Stajić, S., Martinović, A. and Hromiš, N. (2018). Edible offal quality of Swallow-Belly Mangalica pigs reared under an intensive production system – investigation on pigs slaughtered at 100 kg live weight. *Fleischwirtschaft International*, 5: 49-54.

Djekić, I., Škunca, D., Nastasijević, I., Tomović, V. and Tomašević, I. (2018). Transformation of quality aspects throughout the chicken meat supply chain. *British Food Journal*, 120 (5): 1132-50.

Džinić, N., Pezo, L., Radić, N., Šojić, B., Jokanović, M., Tomović, V. and Škaljac, S. (2017). The effects of functional additives on quality characteristics of cooked sausages-mathematical approach. *Romanian Biotechnological Letters*, 22 (5): 12898-906.

Hromiš, N., Šojić, B., Lazić, V., Džinić, N., Mandić, A., Tomović, V., Kravić, S., Škaljac, S., Popović, S. and Šuput, D. (2017). Effect of chitosan coating with the addition of caraway essential oil and beeswax on oxidative stability of petrovská klobása sausage. *Acta Alimentaria*, 46 (3): 361-8.

Jambrec, D., Sakač, M., Jovanov, P., Mišan, A., Pestorić, M., Tomović, V. and Mandić, A. (2016). Effect of processing and cooking on mineral and phytic acid content of buckwheat-enriched tagliatelle. *Chemical Industry and Chemical Engineering Quarterly*, 22 (3): 319-26.

Kocić-Tanackov, S., Blagojev, N., Suturović, I., Dimić, G., Pejin, J., Tomović, V., Šojić, B., Savanović, J., Kravić, S. and Karabasil, N. (2017). Antibacterial activity essential oils against *Escherichia coli*, *Salmonella enterica* and *Listeria monocytogenes*. *Journal of Food Safety and Food Quality*, 68 (4): 88-95.

Lukač, D., Šević, R., Vidović, V., Puvača, N., Tomović, V. and Džinić, N. (2016). Quantitative-genetic analysis of growth intensity of autochthonous breeds Mangalitsa pigs reared in traditional and modern systems. *Thai Journal of Veterinary Medicine*, 46 (3): 409-17.

Lukač, D., Vidović, V., Džinić, N. and Tomović, V. (2016). Phenotypic and genetic analysis of carcass quality of different breeds' fatlings. *Indian Journal of Animal Sciences*, 86 (6): 706-9.

Lukač, D., Vidović, V., Stoisavljević, A., Puvača, N., Džinić, N. and Tomović, V. (2015). Basic chemical composition of meat and carcass quality of fattening hybrids with different slaughter weight. *Hemijska Industrija*, 69, 2, 121-6.

Petrović, J., Rakić, D., Fišteš, A., Pajin, B., Lončarević, I., Tomović, V. and Zarić, D. (2017). Defatted wheat germ application: Influence on cookies' properties with regard to its particle size and dough moisture content. *Food Science and Technology International*, 23 (7): 597-607.

Šević, R., Lukač, D., Vidović, V., Puvača, N., Savić, B., Ljubojević, D., Tomović, V. and Džinić, N. (2017). Neki parametri nutritivnog kvaliteta mesa svinja rase mangulica i landras. *Hemijska Industrija*, 71 (2): 111-8. [Some parameters of nutritional quality of meat obtained from Mangalitsa and Landrace pig breeds. *Hemijska Industrija*, 71 (2): 111-8].

Šojić, B., Tomović, V., Jokanović, M., Ikonić, P., Džinić, N., Kocić-Tanackov, S., Popović, Lj., Tasić, T., Savanović, J. and Živković Šojić N. (2017). Antioxidant activity of *Juniperus communis* L. essential oil in cooked pork sausages. *Czech Journal of Food Science*, 35 (3): 189-93.

Stajić, S., Stanišić, N., Tomović, V., Petričević, M., Stanojković, A., Radović, Č. and Gogić, M. (2017). Farb- und Texturveränderungen während der Lagerung bei Sremska, einer traditionellen serbischen

Macro- and Micromineral Contents in Raw ... 35

Rohwurst. *Fleischwirtschaft*, 8: 103-7. [Changes in colour and texture during storage of Sremska sausage, a traditional Serbian dry-fermented sausage. *Fleischwirtschaft*, 8: 103-7].

Suvajdžić, B., Petronijević, R., Teodorović, V., Tomović, V., Dimitrijević, M., Karabasil, N. and Vasilev, D. (2018). Qualität der Rohwurst Sremski Kulen. *Fleischwirtschaft*, 6: 93-9. [Quality of fermented sausage Sremski Kulen produced under traditional and industrial conditions in Serbia. *Fleischwirtschaft*, 6: 93-9].

Tomašević, I., Tomović, V., Stajić, S., Jokanović, M., Stanišić, N. and Živković, D. (2015). Auswirkungen des schnellen auftauens auf die qualitätsmerkmale von schweinefiletsteaks. *Fleischwirtschaft*, 9: 121-4. [Effects of fast thawing on the quality attributes of pork tenderloin steaks. *Fleischwirtschaft*, 9: 121-4].

Tomović, V., Mastanjević, K., Kovačević, D., Jokanović, M., Kevrešan, Ž., Škaljac, S., Šojić, B., Lukač, D., Škrobot, D. and Despotović. A. (2016). Proximate and mineral composition and cadmium content of main anatomical parts and offal from semi-outdoor reared Black Slavonian pigs. *Agro FOOD Industry Hi Tech*, 27 (6): 39-42.

Tomović, V., Vujadinović, D., Grujić, R., Jokanović, M., Kevrešan, Ž., Škaljac, S., Šojić, B., Tasić, T., Ikonić, P. and Hromiš, N. (2015). Effect of endpoint internal temperature on mineral contents of boiled pork loin. *Journal of Food Processing and Preservation*, 39 (6): 1854-8.

Tomović, V., Vujadinović, D., Grujić, R., Jokanović, M., Kevrešan, Ž., Škaljac, S., Šojić, B., Vasilev, D., Kocić-Tanackov, S. and Hromiš, N. (2016). Auswirkung der Endpunkttemperatur im Inneren auf den Mineralstoffgehalt von Schweinerückenbraten. *Fleischwirtschaft*, 12: 101-5. [Effect of endpoint internal temperature on mineral contents of roasted pork loin. *Fleischwirtschaft*, 12: 101-5].

Tomović, V., Žlender, B., Jokanović, M., Tomović, M., Šojić, B., Škaljac, S., Kevrešan, Ž., Tasić, T., Ikonić, P. and Okanović, Đ. (2016). Physical and chemical characteristics of edible offal from free-range reared Swallow-Belly Mangalica pigs. *Acta Alimentaria*, 45 (2): 190-7.

Tomović, V. M., Jokanović, M. R., Pihler, I. I., Švarc-Gajić, J. V., Vasiljević, I. M., Škaljac, S. B., Šojić, B. B., Živković, D. M., Lukić,

T.B., Despotović, AR. and Tomašević, I. B. (2016). Ultimate pH, colour characteristics and proximate and mineral composition of edible organs, glands and kidney fat from Saanen goat male kids. *Journal of Applied Animal Research*, 45 (1): 430-6.

Tomović, V. M., Šević, R., Jokanović, M., Šojić, B., Škaljac, S., Tasić, T., Ikonić, P., Lušnic Polak, M., Polak, T. and Demšar, L. (2016). Quality traits of longissimus lumborum muscle from White Mangalica, Duroc x White Mangalica and Large White pigs reared under intensive conditions and slaughtered at 150 kg live weight: a comparative study. *Archives Animal Breeding*, 59: 401-415.

Tomović, V. M., Stanišić, N. Z., Jokanović, M. R., Kevrešan, Ž. S., Šojić, B. V., Škaljac, S. B., Tomašević, I. B., Martinović, A. B., Despotović, A.R. and Šuput, D. Z. (2016). Meat quality of Swallow-Belly Mangulica pigs reared under intensive production system and slaughtered at 100 kg live weight. *Hemijska Industrija*, 70 (5): 557-64.

Vasilev, D., Jovetić, M., Vranić, D., Tomović, V., Jokanović, M., Dimitrijević, M., Karabasil, N. and Vasiljević, N. (2016). Qualität und mirkoflora von funktionellen rohwürsten – Untersuchungen von würsten, die mit KCl und CaCl$_2$ als kochsalz-ersatzstoffe hergestellt und mit dem probiotikum *L. casei* LC01 sowie einem präbiotikum angereichert worden sind. *Fleischwirtschaft*, 2: 96-102. [Quality and microflora of functional fermented sausages enriched with probiotic *L. casei* LC01 and prebiotic with KCl and CaCl$_2$ as NaCl substitutes. *Fleischwirtschaft*, 2: 96-102].

Published Papers – In the Journal of National Significance

Džinić, N., Ivić, M., Jokanović, M., Šojić, B., Radić, N., Tomović, V. and Škaljac, S. (2015). Odabrani parametri kvaliteta fino ustinjenih barenih kobasica u tipu viršle sa različitim dodacima. *Uljarstvo*, 46 (1): 65-71. [Selected parameters of quality of hot-dog-type sausages with various additives. *Journal of Edible Oil Industry*, 46 (1): 65-71].

Džinić, N., Ivić, M., Jokanović, M., Šojić, B., Škaljac, S. and Tomović, V. (2016). Chemical, color, texture and sensory properties of čajna kobasica, a dry fermented sausage. *Quality of Life*, 7 (1-2): 5-11.

Macro- and Micromineral Contents in Raw ...   37

Grujić, R., Vujadinović, D., Tomović, V. and Vukić, M. (2015). Uticaj visine temperature i režima toplotne obrade na promijenu tehnoloških osobina mesa. *Hrana u zdravlju i bolesti*, 40 (1): 71-80. [Influence of temperature and heat treatment procedure on the change of technological properties of meat. *Food in Health and Disease*, 40 (1): 71-80].

Hromiš, N., Lazić, V., Šuput, D., Popović, S. and Tomović, V. (2015). Improvement of water vapor barrier properties of chitosan-collagen laminated casings using beeswax. *Analecta Technica Szegedinensia*, 9 (1): 31-8.

Hromiš, N., Šojić, B., Lazić, V., Popović, S., Šuput, D., Bulut, S., Džinić, N., Tomović, V. and Ivić, M. (2018). Two-layer coating based on chitosan for dry fermented sausage preservation. *Journal on Processing and Energy in Agriculture*, 22 (1): 23-6.

Ivić, M., Jokanović, M., Džinić, N., Tomović, V., Škaljac, S., Šojić, B., Peulić, T. and Ikonić, P. (2017). The effect of freezing-thawing and marination time on cooked chicken breast meat quality. *Archives of Veterinary Medicine*, 10 (2): 33-44.

Jokanović, M., Ikonić, P., Škaljac, S., Tasić, T., Tomović, V., Šojić, B., Ivić, M., Petrović, Lj. and Džinić, N. (2017). Proteolysis and texture profile of traditional dry-fermented sausage as affected by primary processing method. *Meat Technology*, 58 (2): 103-9.

Jokanović, M., Tomović, V., Škaljac, S., Šojić, B., Tasić, T., Ikonić, P., Živković, D., Stajić, S., Pajin, B. and Lončarević, I. (2015). Colour and marbling of *M. semimembranosus* and *M. longissimus thoracis et lumborum* from five purebred pigs produced in Vojvodina. *Journal on Processing and Energy in Agriculture*, 19 (1): 48-51.

Lončarević, I., Pajin, B., Petrović, J., Šarac, V., Tomović, V., Zarić, D. and Nikolovski, Z. (2016). Lecitin iz uljane repice kao emulgator u proizvodnji mazivog krem proizvoda. *Uljarstvo*, 47 (1): 47-54. [Rapeseed lecithin as emulsifier in confectionery cream production. *Journal of Edible Oil Industry*, 47 (1): 47-54].

Šojić, B., Džinić, N., Tomović, V., Ikonić, P., Jokanović, M., Kravić, S., Tasić, T. and Škaljac, S. (2016). Effect of starter culture addition on fatty acid profile, oxidative and sensory stability of traditional fermented sausage (petrovská klobása). *Acta Periodica Technologica*, 47: 75-81.

Šojić, B., Hromiš, N., Petrović, Lj., Tomović, V., Mandić, A., Sedej, I., Džinić, N., Lazić, V., Kravić, S. and Škaljac, S. (2015). Effect of packaging method and storage period on fatty acid profile and tbars value of traditional sausage (petrovskà klobàsa). *Journal on Processing and Energy in Agriculture*, 19 (1): 105-7.

Šojić, B., Tomović, V., Džinić, N., Tasić, T., Škaljac, S., Ikonić, P. and Jokanović, M. (2016). Effect of hot and cold deboning meat on the lipid oxidation changes and sensory properties of the traditional sausage *Petrovská klobása*. *Journal on Processing and Energy in Agriculture*, 20 (1): 39-41.

Tasić, T., Ikonić, P., Petrović, Lj., Mandić, A., Škaljac, S., Jokanović, M., Tomović, V., Šojić, B., Ivić, M. and Džinić, N. (2016). Biogenic amines profile of serbian traditional sausage in relation to raw material and production conditions. *Journal of Agricultural Science and Technology B*, 6: 48-56.

Tomašević, I., Đekić, I., Aćimović, M., Stajić, S. and Tomović, V. (2017). The quality difference between frankfurters seasoned with conventional and organic spices. *Acta Periodica Technologica*, 48: 275-84.

Tomašević, I., Tomović, V., Stajić, S., Jokanović, M., Stanišić, N. and Živković, D. (2015). Effects of anatomical location within pork tenderloins on the quality of fast thawed steaks. *Meso*, XVII (5): 455-60.

Tomović, V., Jokanović, M., Kevrešan, Ž., Škaljac, S., Šojić, B., Tasić, T., Ikonić, P., Živković, D., Stajić, S. and Hromiš, N. (2015). Content of macrominerals in the *M. semimembranosus* and *M. longissimus thoracis et lumborum* from five purebred pigs produced in Vojvodina. *Journal on Processing and Energy in Agriculture*, 19 (2): 87-90.

Vujadinović, D., Gojković, V., Vukić, M. and Tomović, V. (2016). Risk analysis for the presence of sodium and phosphates salts in the model systems of organic cooked sausage. *Journal of Hygienic Engineering and Design*, 17: 34-42.

Macro- and Micromineral Contents in Raw ...

Vujadinović, D., Golić, B., Tomović, V., Gojković, V., Vukić, M. and Grujić, R. (2017). Antimicrobial activity of essential oils and fruits supplement in reduced nitrite salts condition. *Matica Srpska Journal for Natural Sciences*, 133: 251-60.

Zekić, V., Džinić, N., Tica, N., Tomović, V. and Milić, D. (2015). Utvrđivanje cene koštanja tradicionalih proizvoda od mesa. *Agroekonomika*, 44 (67): 117-24. [Cost price determination for traditional meat products. *Agrieconomica*, 44 (67): 117-24].

Papers at Scientific Conferences – International Importance

Dzinic, N., Ivic, M., Sojic, B., Jokanovic, M., Tomovic, V., Okanovic, Dj., and Popov Raljic, J. (2015). "Some quality parameters of dry fermented sausages (Čajna kobasica)." Paper presented at the *58th International Meat Industry Conference* (MeatCon2015), 77-80, Zlatibor, Serbia, October, 4-7.

Hromiš, N., Lazić, V., Bulut, S., Popović, S., Šuput, D., Markov, S., Džinić, N., and Tomović, V. (2017). "Influence of beeswax addition on antimicrobial activity of composite chitosan biofilms." Paper presented at the *Fifth international conference sustainable postharvest and food technologies INOPTEP 2017 and XXIX national conference processing and energy in agriculture PTEP* 2017, 138-43, Vršac, Serbia, April 23-28.

Hromiš, N., Lazić, V., Popović, S., Šuput, D., Bulut, S., Džinić, N., Šojić, B., and Tomović, V. (2016). "Two layer chitosan-beeswax coating for application on artificial collagen casings" Paper presented at the FoodTech Congress, III International Congress "*Food Technology, Quality and Safety*," 116-21, Novi Sad, Serbia, October 25-27.

Ikonić, P., Šojić, B., Tasić, T., Jokanović, M., Tomović, V., Škaljac, S., and Novaković, A. (2016). "Comparison of selected physicochemical and sensory properties of traditional fermented sausages produced in Vojvodina (northern Serbia)." Paper presented at the FoodTech Congress, III International Congress "*Food Technology, Quality and Safety,*" 290-5, Novi Sad, Serbia, October, 25-27.

Ikonic, P., Jokanovic, M., Tasic, T., Skaljac, S., Sojic, B., Tomovic, V., Dzinic, N., and Petrovic, Lj. (2015). "The effect of different ripening conditions on proteolysis and texture of dry-fermented sausage Petrovská klobása." Paper presented at the *58ᵗʰ International Meat Industry Conference* (MeatCon2015), 97-100, Zlatibor, Serbia, October 4-7.

Ikonić, P., Tasić, T., Petrović, Lj., Škaljac, S., Jokanović, M., Tomović, V., Šojić, B., and Džinić, N. (2015). "The effect of starter culture on proteolytic changes in traditional fermented sausage petrovska klobasa." Paper presented at the *IV International Congress "Engineering, Ecology and Materials in the Processing Industry,"* 424-31, Jahorina, Bosnia and Herzegovina, March 04-06.

Ivić, M., Džinić, N., Škaljac, S., Jokanović, M., Tomović, V., Šojić, B., Tasić, T., and Ikonić, P. (2017). "Colour and sensory characteristics of traditional dry fermented sausage (Petrovská klobása) as affected by the starter culture." Paper presented at the *V International Congress "Engineering, Environment and Materials in Processing Industry,"* 80-7, Jahorina, Republic of Srpska, Bosnia and Hercegovina, March 15-17.

Ivić, M., Tomović, V., Šević, R., Jokanović, M., Škaljac, S., Džinić, N., Šojić, B., Tasić, T., and Ikonić, P. (2017). "Carcass quality traits of three different pig genotypes, White Mangulica, Duroc × White Mangulica and Large White pigs, reared under intensive conditions and slaughtered at 150 kg live weight." *Paper presented at the 59th International Meat Industry Conference MEATCON2017*, 1-5, Zlatibor, Serbia, October 1-4.

Jokanović, M., Ikonić, B., Ikonić, P., Tomović, V., Tasić, T., Škaljac, S., Šojić, B., Ivić, M., and Džinić, N. (2016). "Application of PCA method for textural properties of three serbian traditional dry fermented sausages." Paper presented at the FoodTech Congress, III International Congress *"Food Technology, Quality and Safety,"* 587-92, Novi Sad, Serbia, October 25-27.

Jokanović, M., Ikonić, P., Tomović, V., Škaljac, S., Šojić, B., Tasić, T., Ivić, M., and Džinić, N. (2017). "Texture characteristics of serbian traditional dry fermented sausage as effected by production process." Paper presented at the *V International Congress "Engineering, Environment and Materials in Processing Industry*," 161-6, Jahorina, Republic of Srpska, Bosnia and Hercegovina, March 15-17.

Jokanović, M., Ikonić, P., Tasić, T., Tomović, V., Šojić, B., Škaljac, S., Džinić, N., and Novaković, A. (2015). "Comparison of the texture profile characteristics of two serbian traditional dry fermented sausages." Paper presented at the *IV International Congress "Engineering, Ecology and Materials in the Processing Industry*," 662-6, Jahorina, Bosnia and Herzegovina, March 04-06.

Jokanović, M., Tomović, V., Škaljac, S., Šojić, B., Tasić, T., Ikonić, P., Živković, D., Stajić, S., Pajin, B., and Lončarević, I. (2015). "Effect of bred and muscle type on colour and marbling of pork produced in Vojvodina." Paper presented at the *Fourth international conference sustainable postharvest and food technologies INOPTEP 2015 and XXVII national conference processing and energy in agriculture PTEP 2015*, 81-5, Divčibare, Serbia, April 19-24.

Škaljac, S., Petrović, Lj. Jokanović, M., Tomović, V., Ivić, M., Tasić, T., Ikonić, P., Šojić, B., and Džinić, N. (2017). "The influence of smoking on colour and content of polycyclic aromatic hydrocarbons in dry fermented sausages (Petrovská klobása)." Paper presented at the *V International Congress "Engineering, Environment and Materials in Processing Industry*," 136-44, Jahorina, Republic of Srpska, Bosnia and Hercegovina, March 15-17.

Škaljac, S., Petrović, Lj., Jokanović, M., Tomović, V., Tasić, T., Ivić, M., Šojić, B., Ikonić, P., and Džinić, N. (2017). "The influence of smoking in traditional conditions on content of polycyclic aromatic hydrocarbons in Petrovská klobása." Paper presented at the *59th International Meat Industry Conference MEATCON2017*, 1-5, Zlatibor, Serbia, October 1-4.

Šojić, B., Džinić, N., Tomović, V., Ikonić, P., Jokanović, M., Tasić, T., Škaljac, S., and Ivić, M. (2016). "Effect of starter culture addition on oxidative stability of fermented sausage produced in traditional manner." Paper presented at the FoodTech Congress, III International Congress "*Food Technology, Quality and Safety*," 671-88, Novi Sad, Serbia, October, 25-27.

Sojic, B., Dzinic, N., Tomovic, V., Jokanovic, M., Ikonic, P., Tasic, T., Skaljac, S., Danilovic, B., and Ivic, M. (2015). "Effect of the addition of Staphylococus xylosus on the oxidative stabilitty of traditional sausage (Petrovská klobása)." **Paper presented at the** *58th International Meat Industry Conference* (MeatCon2015), 262-5, Zlatibor, Serbia, October 4-7.

Šojić, B., Hromiš, N., Petrović, Lj., Tomović, V., Mandić, A., Sedej, I., Džinić, N., Lazić, V., Kravić, S., and Škaljac, S. (2015). "Effect of packaging method on tbars value and sensory properties of traditional sausage (petrovskà klobàsa)." **Paper presented at the** *Fourth international conference sustainable postharvest and food technologies INOPTEP 2015 and XXVII national conference processing and energy in agriculture PTEP* 2015, 230-5, Divčibare, Serbia, April 19-24.

Šojić, B., Ikonić, P., Pavlić, B., Zeković, Z., Tomović, V., Kocić-Tanackov, S., Džinić, N. Škaljac, S., Ivić, M., Jokanović, M., and Tasić, T. (2017). "The effect of essential oil from sage (*Salvia officinalis* L.) herbal dust (food industry by-product) on the microbiological stability of fresh pork sausages." *Paper presented at the 59th International Meat Industry Conference MEATCON2017*, 1-5, Zlatibor, Serbia, October 1-4.

Šojić, B., Tomović, V., Džinić, N., Savanović, J., and Savanović, D. (2016). *"Effect of caraway essential oil on pork cooked sausage quality."* Paper presented at *the XI Conference of Chemists, Technologists and Environmentalists of Republic of Srpska*, 295-9, Teslić, Bosnia and Herzegovina, November 18-19.

Stanišić, N., Stanojković, A., Tomović, V., Petričević, M., Živković, V., Gogić, M., and Radović, Č. (2016). "Textural and colour changes through the one year storage of dry fermented Sremska sausage manufactured with different pork fat levels." Paper presented at the *Second International Symposium of Veterinary Medicine (ISVM2016),* 283-90, Belgrade, Serbia, June 22-24.

Tasic, T., Ikonic, P., Jokanovic, M., Mandic, A., Tomovic, V., Sojic, B., and Skaljac, S. (2015). "Content of vasoactive amines in Sremski kulen and Sremska kobasica traditional dry fermented sausages from Vojvodina."

Paper presented at the *58th International Meat Industry Conference* (MeatCon2015), 282-4, Zlatibor, Serbia, October 4-7.

Tomašević, I., Stajić, S., Aćimović, M., Škunca, D., Tomović, V., and Đekić, I. (2016). "Garlic powder promotes lipid oxidation in frankfurters." Paper presented at the *62nd ICoMST - International Congress of Meat Science and Technology – Meat for Global Sustainability*, Bangkok, Thailand, August 14-19.

Tomović, V., Jokanović, M., Kevrešan, Ž., Šojić, B., Škaljac, S., Tasić, T., Ikonić, P., Živković, D., Stajić, S., and Lončarević, I. (2015). "Content of microminerals in the *M. semimembranosus* and *M. longissimus thoracis et lumborum* from pigs produced in Vojvodina." Paper presented at the IV International Congress *"Engineering, Ecology and Materials in the Processing Industry*," 432-7, Jahorina, Bosnia and Herzegovina, March 04-06.

Tomović, V., Jokanović, M., Kevrešan, Ž., Škaljac, S., Šojić, B., Tasić, T., Ikonić, P., Živković, D., Stajić, S., and Hromiš, N. (2015). "Effect of bred and muscle type on macrominerals content of pork produced in Vojvodina." Paper presented at the *Fourth international conference sustainable postharvest and food technologies INOPTEP 2015 and XXVII national conference processing and energy in agriculture PTEP 2015*, 274-9, Divčibare, Serbia, April 19-24.

Tomovic, V., Jokanovic, M., Pihler, I., Vasiljevic, I., Skaljac, S., Sojic, B., Tomasevic, I., Tomovic, M., Martinovic, A., and Lukac, D. (2015). "Cadmium levels of edible offal from Saanen goat male kids" Paper presented at the *58th International Meat Industry Conference* (MeatCon2015), 289-92, Zlatibor, Serbia, October 4-7.

In: Pork Consumption and Health
Editor: Frank L. Moore

ISBN: 978-1-53614-991-3
© 2019 Nova Science Publishers, Inc.

Chapter 2

PORK FOODBORNE PARASITES OF PUBLIC HEALTH INTEREST IN MEXICO

I. B. Hernandez-Cortazar[1], PhD, E. Guzman-Marin[1], PhD, K. Y. Acosta-Viana[1], PhD, A. Ortega-Pacheco[2], PhD, J. I. Chan-Perez[1], PhD and M. Jimenez-Coello[1,], PhD*

[1]Centro de Investigaciones Regionales "Dr Hideyo Noguchi," Autonomous University of Yucatan, Merida Yucatan, Mexico
[2]Facultad de Medicina Veterinaria y Zootecnia, Autonomous University of Yucatan, Merida Yucatan, Mexico

ABSTRACT

The ingestion of raw or undercooked pork poses a public health risk, since pork is the main transmitter of parasites, which include the protozoa *Toxoplasma gondii* (*T. gondii*) and the helminths *Trichinella spiralis* (*T. spiralis*) and *Taenia solium (T. solium)*. These three 'T' porkborne parasites have been responsible for most of the porkborne illnesses

---

[*] Corresponding Author E-mail: mjcoello@correo.uady.mx.

throughout history; they are still endemic, and therefore are important public-health concerns, in developing countries. In Mexico, these three 'T' porkborne parasites are considered re-emerging parasites, and they represents a risk for the population that consumes large quantities of pork. Currently, inspection procedures are effective in eliminating the majority of the risks from *T. spiralis* and *T. solium* in certified slaughterhouses, due to the training of inspectors in the detection of tissue cysts. However, there are still clandestine slaughterhouses that do not have adequate surveillance methods to identify these parasites. Furthermore, for *T. gondii* no suitable methods for post-slaughter detection are available, where intervention measures at the animal level may be key to successful prevention. Early detection of the parasite is not easy, and the implementation of molecular techniques must be improved and made available mainly in endemic areas, in order to establish an accurate diagnosis, because isolation procedures are long, more expensive and often not sufficiently sensitive. The objectives of this chapter are to describe the epidemiological situation of these three parasites transmitted by pork in Mexico, outline the main lines of prevention, and describe the molecular methods that can be used for the early and accurate detection.

Keywords: pig-meat, zoonosis, parasites, Mexico, molecular detection, prevention

1. INTRODUCTION

Foodborne zoonoses have been estimated to annually affect 10% of the global population, among which zoonotic parasites constitute an important class of aetiological agents [1]. Foodborne parasites are expected to have a strong impact on public health in the future, particularly with the increase in meat consumption that is taking place in the world and the recognition that billions of people lack basic water services [2]. Pork is one of the main transmitters of parasites that include the protozoa *Toxoplasma gondii* (*T. gondii*) and the helminths *Trichinella spiralis* (*T. spiralis*) and *Taenia solium* (*T. solium*). These three 'T' parasites have been responsible for most porkborne illnesses throughout history; they are still endemic, and therefore are important public health concerns, in developing countries [1]. They are important because pork has long been the most consumed meat globally, and the projections of the future global pork demand remain robust [3]. The disability adjusted life-years (DALYs) have been estimated for human cysticercosis, toxoplasmosis and trichinellosis, with 2.78 million DALYs (95% UI 2.14–3.61 million), 825,000 DALYs (95% UI 561,000–1.26 million) and 550 (95% UI 285–934), respectively [4]. The United States has improved demonstrably over recent decades in pork safety due to the changes in swine production methods. The implementation of intensive confinement production systems has eliminated the risk of foodborne parasites [5]. The environment in which animals are kept determines the course and severity of disease expression; a highly contaminated environment for animals with a weakened immune system often tips the balance and makes a disease clinical [6]. The potential sources of infection at the farm level for these three parasites include water, feed, soil/organic material contaminated with oocysts or eggs, feed contaminated with infected animal tissue, and exposure to and ingestion of tissue from rodents, pigs, or wildlife carcasses [7]. The culinary preferences for fresh, slightly cooked, and ready-to-eat food and the increasing demands for meat in developing countries are increasing the risks posed by foodborne parasites [8]. In addition, pigs raised in outdoor systems inherently confront higher risks of exposure to foodborne parasites, particularly *T. gondii* [5].

Several endemic countries (such as some countries in Asia, Eastern Europe, and South America) cannot avoid human infection due to inadequate quality control in meat production [2]. In México, reporting the ocurrence of these three parasites is considered mandatory by monthly notification to the official dependencies of animal health of the country [9]. According to the Mexican regulation (NOM-SSA1-2004), pork must be free of *Trichinella spiralis*, *Taenia solium* and other parasites; however, trichinoscopy is not mandatory [10]. Regarding, *T. gondii*, there are no official regulations that required the identification of tissue cysts in the carcasses. In the country, the Federal Inspection Type Certification, (abbreviated TIF), is an acknowledgment granted by SAGARPA (Secretary of Agriculture, Livestock, Rural Development, Fisheries and Food), that performs a thorough inspection procedure and supervises and traces industrial establishments that are dedicated to produce, store, sacrifice, process and distribute all kinds of meats and their derivatives. The TIF recognition opens the possibility of international trade, since these establishments are the only ones eligible to export. Currently, in Mexico there are 457 TIF slaughterhouses where the surveillance of the meat is guaranteed [11]. However, in local markets in the central region of Mexico, it has been reported that 11.3% of the meat sold comes from pigs raised at home, which are illegally slaughtered [12]. In rural regions of Mexico, it is common to raise backyard pigs without adequate sanitary conditions, and these animals are slaughtered in unhealthy facilities that are not inspected for pathogens that may be encysted in the animal tissues. Unfortunately, there is no record of the illegal slaughterhouses established in Mexico, where proper inspection of the pig carcasses is not carried out, representing a risk for consumers. In addition, it has been shown that methods of direct observation of meat have low sensitivity, so the frequency of these porkborne parasites in Mexico may be underestimated [13]. Efforts to maintain innocuous pork meat ensure that the population is free to acquire these parasitic infections. The implementation of efficient, accessible, and controllable inspection policies for livestock, slaughterhouses, and meat processing and packaging companies is highly recommended [14].

In this chapter, we present epidemiological data reported for these three "T" pork parasites of public health interest in Mexico. Additionally, we described the main molecular methods used for the detection of these parasites in pork meat, as well as the prevention measures.

2. Methods

2.2. Epidemiology of *Taenia solium*

Taenia solium is a hermaphrodite cestode parasite that infects humans and pigs. Worldwide, it is estimated that approximately 2 to 3 million people are infected with *T. solium*, and it is thought that some 50,000 people die annually from this parasitosis due to complications in the nervous system or heart failure [15]. *T. solium* is endemic in tropical regions of the world (Latin

Pork Foodborne Parasites of Public Health Interest in Mexico 49

America, Southeast Asia and Africa). Normally, the cycle life of *T. solium* involves two hosts (human and pig) in which this parasite completes its life cycle. The disease is known as taeniasis and is more common in rural communities where domestic pigs are raised under free conditions, allowed to roam in the backyards and feed on fecal matter deposited by people in backyards because of a lack of sanitary infrastructure [15, 16]. Humans become infected by *T. solium* when eating inadequately cooked pork that contains the larvae. Once consumed, the larvae restart their development to the adult forms in the small intestine of humans, specifically the duodenum (5 to 12 weeks of patency). *T. solium* attach to the wall of the small intestine using the scolex armed with 4 suckers and 2 rows of large and small hooks [15, 16, 17]. Each segment or proglottids of *T. solium* have different degrees of development (immature, mature and gravid). The last segments are called gravid proglottids that contain infective eggs; these segments detach from the strobila (the main body of the parasite) and are shed in the environment through the feces. Adult *T. solium* can eliminate up to 300,000 eggs per day. These segments remain active and show movements. *T. solium* could reach 2 to 7 meters in length and live less than 5 years but occasionally could persist nearly 25 years. The infection of adults with *T. solium* is often asymptomatic, but the presence in many adults can cause mucosal irritation, abdominal pain, diarrhea, constipation, weight loss and obstruction of the intestinal lumen [15, 16, 17].

The natural intermediate host for *T. solium* is the pig; however, the parasite can occasionally be found in dogs, cats, sheep, camels, monkeys and humans (Figure 1, *Life cycle image courtesy of DPDx*) [18]. Pigs are infected through the consumption of the eggs of *T. solium* scattered by wind or rain that contaminate the water or their food. In the interior of the host, the embryo is activated and leaves the egg, penetrates the intestinal mucosa, enters blood circulation and disperses to other tissues between 24 and 72 hours after ingestion [15, 18]. Once in the tissue, the embryo is transformed into cysticerci with the shape of an ovoid vesicle [18]. In the pig, the cysticercus is located in the striated or cardiac muscle. In humans, cysticerci can invade different types of muscle (striated and cardiac), the central nervous system (brain), the subcutaneous tissue and other tissues of the host, such as the liver, lugs, abdominal cavity and eye orbit [15, 18]. The most common cases of cysticercosis in humans aredetected in the central nervous system. The presence of cysticerci in the tissue unchains many mechanisms in the human body such as inflammation, fibrosis and some calcification. In the brain, this immunological reaction produces neurological signs such as epilepsy, seizures, headaches, nausea, visual disturbance, focal weakness, and paresthesias. The neurological form of the disease is called neurocysticercosis and is the most serious form of the disease [18, 19]. Regardless of the source of the infection, the lack of hygienic habits, such as washing hands after going to the bathroom and before consuming meals, are the main reasons for the presentation of cysticercosis in humans (Taenia and Cysti). Other factors, such as the use of wastewater for irrigation or the consumption of contaminated water from rivers, could contribute to the spread of the eggs [18].

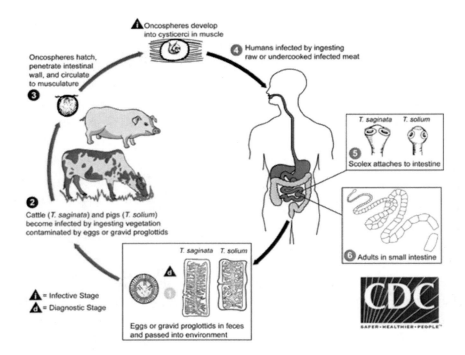

Figure 1. Life cycle of Taenia spp (image courtesy of DPDx) www.cdc.gov/parasites/(https://www.cdc.gov/parasites/).

Pork Foodborne Parasites of Public Health Interest in Mexico 51

Table 1. Studies of *Taenia solium* in pigs from Mexico

Taenia solium					
Sample	**Origin**	**Assay**	**Positivity**	**State**	**Reference**
Tongue	Backyard	Direct palpation	25%	Hidalgo	[23]
Tongue	Backyard	Direct palpation	4%	Morelos	[24]
Tongue	Backyard	Direct palpation	6.5%	Michoacán	[28]
Tongue	Backyard	Direct palpation	2.6%	Morelos	[25]
Serum		Western Blot	5.2%		
Serum	Backyard	Western Blot	23%	Yucatan	[20]
	Semi intensive		25%		
	Intensive reared		2%		
Serum	Backyard	Western Blot	35%	Yucatan	[21]
Tongue		Direct palpation	23%		
Serum	Backyard	Western blot	29%	Yucatan	[22]
Tongue	Backyard	Direct palpation	13.3%	Morelos	[26]
Tongue	Backyard	Direct palpation	7%	Guerrero	[29]
Body		Ultrasound	3.6%		
Serum		ELISA	17.7%		
Serum	Backyard	ELISA	19.0%	Morelos	[27]

2.2.1. Taenia solium in Pigs in Mexico

In Mexico, the epidemiological studies that have focused on binomial taeniasis/cysticercosis in humans. However, most of studies were conducted prior to the year 2000. At the national level, the actual prevalence of this parasitosis associated with poverty conditions is still unknown. Many of the existing studies carried out in Mexico have been isolated, focusing on some states, and few have jointly evaluated the positivity of people and pigs. Table 1 shows the results of different studies in which infection by *T. solium* cysticerci was diagnosed in pigs reared in rural communities in Mexico. The highest prevalence of pigs infected by cysticerci was found in pigs from Yucatán State (southeast region), with a prevalence of 23 to 35% [20, 21, 22]. In central Mexico, a prevalence of 25% was reporteed from Hidalgo State [23] and 2.6% to 13.3% was reported for the state of Morelos [24, 25, 26, 27]. For the Pacific coast, prevalence rates of 6.5% and 17.7% were reported for Michoacan and Guerrero State, respectively [28, 29]. In Mexico it is estimated that 2.1 million pigs live in rural areas, inside backyard systems [30]. Considering the percentage of infected pigs in some studies

52 I.B. Hernandez-Cortazar, E. Guzman-Marin, K.Y. Acosta-Viana et al.

conducted in the country, the risk of acquiring taeniasis and cysticercosis is high.

Approximately, 4,328 cases of human cystcercosis have been reported between 2000 and 2010 [31]. Recently, in 2017, 227 and 179 cases of Taeniasis and Cysticercosis have been reported, respectively. In the January-October period of 2018, 139 cases of Taeniasis and 187 cases of Cysticercosis have been reported [32]. The persistence of cases diagnosed in humans in different states of the country suggests that the prevalence of this disease in pigs reared in backyards could be underestimated. In Mexico, the lack of sanitary infrastructure, the availability of decent housing with latrines, the low economic income of families in rural communities, the backyard rising of animals for self-consumption and the saturation of health centers contribute to the persistence of this parasitosis.

2.3. Epidemiology of *Toxoplasma gondii*

Toxoplasma gondii is an apicomplexan protozoan intracellular parasite with a widespread distribution in both developed and developing countries [33]. *T. gondii* has veterinary and medical importance, because it may cause abortion or congenital disease in its intermediate hosts [34]. Additionally, *T. gondii* can cause severe illness in immunocompromised individuals [35], and ocular toxoplasmosis is frequently observed in immunocompetent patients [36]. Felids are the only definitive hosts in which the parasite can complete its sexual cycle and spread millions of oocysts into the environment. Although the number of oocysts produced is a key element in environmental contamination and consequently in parasite transmission, *T. gondii* is also able to rely on its asexual cycle in all warm-blooded animals (mammals and birds) and humans [35]. Initial infection of a host is usually accomplished by the rapidly replicating form of the organism called tachyzoites. However, in an immune competent host following the activation of the immune system, the tachyzoites undergo a conversion to the slowly replicating form of the organism called bradyzoites, which cluster to form tissue cysts. These tissue cysts can persist in the brain and other organs for extended periods of time without the generation of an apparent immune response. At various times, a portion of these tissue cysts can reactivate into tachyzoites and, if the immune response is adequate, subsequently reconvert into bradyzoites containing tissue cysts. Through these interconversions, *T. gondii* can establish life-long persistence in immune competent hosts [33].

There are two major modes of transmission of *T. gondii*: infection may occur by the ingestion of food or water contaminated with oocysts excreted by infected cats or by ingesting uncooked or undercooked meat containing tissue cysts (Figure 2, *Life cycle image courtesy of DPDx*). The proportion of the human population that acquires an infection by the ingestion of oocysts in the environment or by eating contaminated meat is not known, and there are no tests available that can determine the infection source. However, sero-epidemiologic data suggest that ingesting improperly cooked meat containing *T. gondii* is a major source of infection for humans in the United States [37, 38]. In addition, pregnant women in Europe identified meat ingestion as the major source of *T. gondii* infection (30–63% of cases) [39].

It has been reported that in meat-producing animals, tissue cysts of *T. gondii* are most frequently observed in these tissues of infected pigs, sheep, and goats, and are less frequently in infected poultry, rabbits, dogs, and horses, with pork being the major source of *T. gondii* infection [34]. These animals harbor tissue cysts, and human consumers can be infected by ingestion of these cysts in raw or undercooked meat [40]. Virtually all edible portions of an animal can harbor viable *T. gondii* tissue cysts [41], and tissue cysts can survive in food animals for years [40]. It has been shown that a single *T. gondii* oocyst is capable of producing an infection in pigs, and among the most parasitized organs with tissue cysts are the tongue, brain and heart [42].

The reduction of the risk of *T. gondii* infections in pigs is possible, using intensive farm management with adequate measures of hygiene, confinement, and prevention [34]. In contrast, pigs reared on organic farms have shown to have a higher *T. gondii* prevalence than pigs from conventional farms [35].

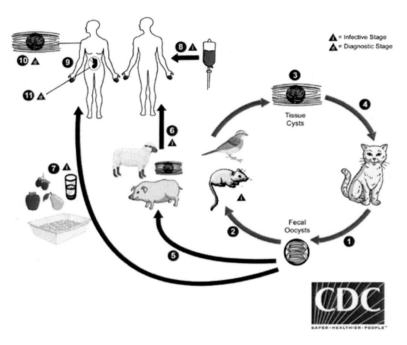

Figure 2. Life cycle of Toxoplasma gondii (image courtesy of DPDx) www.cdc.gov/parasites/(https://www.cdc.gov/parasites/).

2.3.1. Toxoplasma gondii in Pigs in Mexico

In Mexico, there are few studies of *T. gondii* carried out in pigs, and most of the studies have searched for antibodies against the parasite, which only indicate exposure (Table 2). However, the molecular detection of *T. gondii* in pork has been poorly studied. For a better analysis of the studies of *T. gondii* in pigs for consumption in Mexico, the country was divided by geographical region (north, center and south), and a great diversity of climatic conditions was found between these regions that could influence the survival of the *T. gondii* parasite.

In the north region, Durango State (northwest) reported a seroprevalence of 9.1% in pigs raised in backyards and Sonora State (northwest end and limits to the north with the USA), showed a seroprevelence of 16% [43]. In Baja California Sur State (northwestern), characterized as having a desert climate, a prevalence of 13% was found in domestic pigs at slaughter [44].

Table 2. Studies of *Toxoplasma gondii* in pigs from Mexico

Toxoplasma gondii					
Sample	**Origin**	**Assay**	**Positivity**	**State**	**Reference**
Serum	Abattoir	ELISA	IgG 8.9%	Morelos	[45]
Muscle	Butcher shops	Bioassay	IgG 2.1%	Jalisco	[46]
Serum	Farms with cats	ELISA	IgG 100%	Yucatán	[48]
Serum	Backyard ND	MAT	IgG 16% IgG 9.1%	Durango Sonora	[43]
Serum	Backyard Farm	MAT	IgG 17.2% IgG 0.5%	Oaxaca	[53]
Serum Blood	Farm	ELISA PCR	IgM 92.5% IgG 95.8% DNA 50.8%	Yucatán	[49]
Serum	Backyard	ELISA	IgG 75%	Yucatán	[50]
Serum	Backyard	MAT	IgG 45.3%	Veracruz	[47]
Serum	Backyard	MAT	IgG 13%	Baja California	[44]
Serum Tongue Loin	Backyard	ELISA nPCR	IgG 96.6% Tongue 23.21% Loin 7%	Yucatán	[51]
Serum Tissue	Semi-extensive breeding	ELISA qPCR	IgG 53% DNA 5.3%	Yucatán	[52]

ND: Not data.

The first report of *T. gondii* in pigs in Mexico was in the central region, where they analyzed 6 to 10-month-old pigs weighing 90-100 kg from an abattoir of Morelos State, and they found a prevalence of 8.9% using ELISA [45]. Another study conducted in Jalisco State (west region that borders the Pacific Ocean), they analyzed 48 pork samples from butcher shops and found that all the samples were negative by histology and by PCR; however, a positivity of antibodies against *T. gondii* of 2.1% in pork meat was detected through bioassay [46]. In Veracruz State (eastern region and the coastline on the Gulf of Mexico) a seroprevalence of 45.3% was reported in domestic pigs raised in backyards using the Microscopic Agglutination Test (MAT), showing that a tropical-humid climate, feeding with leftovers, storing pig food in the owner's home, and free ranging was associated with *T. gondii* seropositivity in pigs [47].

In the southern region, the Yucatan State (northern part of the Yucatan peninsula) has carried out the largest number of studies of *T. gondii* in these animals, finding high seroprevalences in pigs reared on farms as well as pigs reared in backyards. A study in this region analyzed the infection dynamics of *T. gondii* in two fattening pig farms exposed to high and low cat densities and found that 100% of finished pigs had contact with the *T. gondii* regardless of the relative density of the cats [48]. Another study in Yucatan, reported a positivity of *T. gondii* DNA in 50.8% of the blood samples and a seroprevalence of 96% in pigs reared on farms, indicating a high circulation of the parasite [49]. In addition, backyard pigs have reported seroprevalences of 75% from the same region [50]. The high circulation of *T. gondii* in pigs intended for human consumption in Yucatan has led to investigations of the presence of DNA in pork using PCR. Regarding the presence of the parasite in pork, the first report in the southeast of Mexico found a positivity through an nPCR of 23.2% and 7% for samples of tongue and loin tissue, respectively [51]. Subsequently, the parasitic burden of *T. gondii* in Mexican hairless pig (Sus scrofa) tissues using quantitative real-time PCR (qPCR) was determined, finding a positivity of 5.3% of the tissue samples with an average of 2.5 ± 2.71, 0.26 ± 0.39 and 0.31 ± 0.37 parasites per gram for the leg muscle, heart and tongue tissue, respectively [52]. In Oaxaca State, a seroprevalence in pigs raised in backyards of 17.2% and in pigs raised on farms of 0.5% was reported, confirming that the management system (outdoor *vs.* indoor with biosecurity) is a key factor in the epidemiology of swine toxoplasmosis [53]. The relevance between these studies is that the southern region is endemic to toxoplasmosis, with a high prevalence in the human population and in different animal species [54].

2.4. Epidemiology of *Trichinella spiralis*

Trichinella is one of the most widespread parasites infecting people and other mammals all over the world in most climates, except for deserts [55]. Trichinellosis infection follows the ingestion of raw or undercooked meat containing *Trichinella* larvae [56], mainly from pigs, wild boar or horses

Pork Foodborne Parasites of Public Health Interest in Mexico   57

[57, 58]. *Trichinella spiralis* (*T. spiralis*) has a cosmopolitan distribution, and it affects domestic and wild mammals [59]. In Central and South America, the etiological agent of human trichinellosis has been reported to be *T. spiralis*; however, only in a few cases has the parasite species been properly identified [60]. Its clinical manifestations are not specific; thus, the diagnosis of trichinellosis is not easy to make [61]. The life cycle begins when the larvae are released after gastric digestion and mature into adult worms that penetrate the mucosa of the intestine. After fertilization, the female sheds new larvae that disseminate throughout the host to find their definitive location, the striated muscle, where they encyst. This larval migration may result in severe lesions, particularly when larvae migrate to the heart or the brain [55]. Encystment is completed in 4 to 5 weeks, and the encysted larvae may remain viable for several years. Ingestion of the encysted larvae perpetuates the cycle. Rats and rodents are primarily responsible for maintaining the endemicity of this infection. Carnivorous/omnivorous animals, such as pigs or bears, feed on infected rodents or meat from other animals (Image 3, *Life cycle image courtesy of DPDx*).

Worldwide, data from 1986 to 2009 implicated domestic pigs as the major source of infection (53%) in outbreaks [62], most of them in Eastern Europe and Argentina, where the traditional small, "backyard" rearing of pigs for household and local use often involve high risk rearing practices, especially the feeding of food waste. Although commercially produced pork under controlled management now accounts for approximately half of the world's pork production, the demand by consumers, especially in Europe and North America, for free-range pork is increasing [63]. In addition, Trichinellosis is common in some rural areas of South America and Asia but is quite infrequent in urban regions [55]. In Mexico, 453 human cases of trichinosis have been reported from 1893 to 1995, which were confirmed by the finding of larval *T. spiralis* in diaphragm tissue. Chihuahua State, have been reported the largest outbreak in humans, which was associated with the consumption of pork sausage, even though the anatomical parts of the infected animals presented health check seals [64].

In pigs, very few studies have found pigs infected with *T. spiralis*; however, these data are not reliable since they have not been investigated in other states of the country, especially in production systems with unsanitary conditions [65]. Despite the scarcity of studies on *T. spiralis*, so far in 2018, there have been 9 cases of trichinosis in the human population in Mexico [32]. In rural areas of Mexico, it is common to have pigs as part of the family economy. Unfortunately, pigs are left to breed freely, and they go where they can find food, which is in spaces where there is garbage and the presence of the domestic rat, which is part of the transmission cycle of this parasite (rat-pig-human) [66]. In addition, the clandestine slaughter of backyard animals is frequent [67].

2.4.1. Trichinella spiralis in Pigs in Mexico

Most of the studies on pigs are very old. In a review, from 1909 to 1999 there was a positivity of 0-6% of *T. spiralis* in pig carcasses, mainly from trichinoscopy and artificial digestion techniques. In 1989, samples from backyard pigs were analyzed by ELISA, and seroprevalences of <1%, 14% and 24% were found for the state of Michoacan, Veracruz and the State of Mexico, respectively [68]. However, there have been few states where these investigations have been made, mainly in Mexico City, the State of Mexico, Tamaulipas, Jalisco, Sonora, Michoacan, Veracruz and Zacatecas [60]. Recent epidemiological studies of *T. spiralis* in pigs are scarce, which could contribute to an underestimation of the occurrence of this parasite in pigs destined for consumption, especially those that are reared in backyards and do not have adequate sanitary conditions, representing a risk for consumers. The few studies that have been conducted on *T. spiralis* in pigs are located in the center of the country (Table 3). One of the studies that analyzed pork samples from butchers and local markets, found all the negative samples through trichinoscopy [69]. Another study, used serological tests (ELISA and Western blot) and found a seroprevalence of 12.4% in farm and backyard pigs [70]. The last report we have analyzed samples of pork sausage, finding a positivity of 3.4 and 4% by artificial digestion and by trichinoscopy, respectively [65].

Table 3. Studies of *Trichinella spiralis* in pigs from Mexico from the year 2000 to date

Trichinella spiralis					
Sample	**Origin**	**Assay**	**Positivity**	**State**	**Reference**
Pork	Butcher Public market Ambulatory market	Trichinoscopy	0%	Distrito Federal	[69]
Serum	Farm/ Backyard	ELISA/WB	12.4%	State of Mexico	[70]
Chop sausage	ND	Artificial digestion Trichinoscopy	3.4% 4%	State of Mexico Michoacán Hidalgo Morelos	[65]

ND. Not data.

2.5. Diagnostic Methods for the Detection of Pork Parasites

2.5.1. Diagnostic Methods of Taenia solium in Pork

At the field level, several detection methods of *T. solium* in pigs are used, including the following: 1) Palpation. Tactile inspection is made in search of cysticerci in the body of the pigs and can be performed before the animals are slaughtered. This method consists of palpating the surface of the tongue to determine the presence of nodules of *T. solium* cysticerci. It has been reported that this method has a sensitivity of 70% and a specificity of 100% [71]. 2) Direct observation. Direct inspection of organs and pig carcasses in search of cysticerci and is carried out during the slaughter stage of animals at certified slaughterhouses. This inspection is carried out by trained veterinary personnel for this purpose [29]. 3) ELISA and Western blot. These techniques allow the detection of antibodies against *T. solium* in samples of serum from pigs. The Western blot technique is commonly used as a confirmatory test due to its high sensitivity (97%) and specificity (100%) [72]. The ELISA demonstrated a sensitivity of 83.7 to 86% and a specificity of 95.7 to 95.9% [73]. 4) Ultrasound. This method consists of

60 *I.B. Hernandez-Cortazar, E. Guzman-Marin, K.Y. Acosta-Viana et al.*

observing the presence of cysticerci through portable ultrasound equipment by examining the anatomical regions where cysticerci is located, offering greater sensitivity than visual inspection and palpation. This technique can be applied in both live animals and animal carcasses [74].

2.5.2. Diagnostic Methods of Toxoplasma gondii in Pork

In Mexico, *T. gondii* is not among the mandatory inspection diseases in slaughterhouses. However, the main diagnostic tests for this agent are the following: 1) Serology. This method allows for the detection of antibodies in animals. Among the serological tests used for the rapid diagnosis of toxoplasmosis there is an ELISA and MAT. In addition, Western blot (sensitivity of 84.7% and a specificity of 96.7%) [75] and the Indirect immunofluorescent antibody test (IFAT) could be employed to diagnose of this disease [76]. The latter has been used with a cut-off point of 1:64 and in the 80% of the positive cases, and it has been possible to isolate *T. gondii* by inoculation in mice [77]. Currently, there are commercial ELISA kits for the detection of antibodies against *T. gondii* in porcine serum samples [78]. With respect to the detection of *T. gondii* in pork samples, the MAT has been proposed for examining tissue fluid and has had good results for detection [79]. 2) Molecular biology. With respect to molecular diagnosis, PCR variants have been developed as a real-time PCR, PCR point for the detection of *T. gondii* in blood and tissue samples [80] and nested PCR [81]. In addition, a protocol that includes the magnetic capture of *T. gondii* DNA and a real-time PCR have been developed, which examine large samples of pork (100g) with a limit of detection of 230 taquizoites, and this method has been validated by ISO 17025 certification [82, 83].

2.5.3. Diagnostic Methods of Trichinella spiralis in Pork

The main techniques used for the detection of *T. spiralis* in pork are the following: 1) Trichinoscopy. This involves examining a sample of tissue in which the cystic form of the parasite is observed placed between two sheets of glass under a microscope. This method is applied in the slaughterhouses but show low sensitivity when parasitic loads are less than 2 larvae per gram of meat [84]. 2) Artificial Digestion. This technique consists of dissolving the muscle tissue using pepsin, protease and hydrochloric acid to detect the encysted larvae of *T. spiralis*. Currently, there is a commercial kit for this purpose (PrioCHECK™ Trichinella AAD Kit) that complies with international standards and produces a faster and less risky digestion for operators compared to the conventional method [85]. 3) Serological tests. ELISA assays and immunochromatography have been developed and applied in research but not for field-level diagnosis. However, these tests have been effective for the detection of *T. spirals* in natural and artificially infected pigs [86, 87]. 4) Molecular biology. As in other infectious agents, there are protocols to perform conventional PCR, real-time PCR and loop mediation isothermal amplification to detect *T. spiralis* in naturally infected wild and domestic pigs [88, 89].

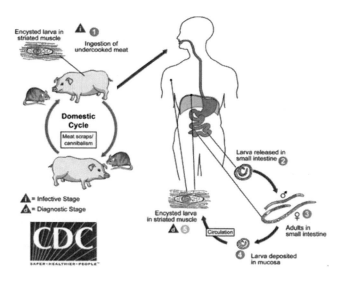

Figure 3. Life cycle of *Trichinella spiralis* (image courtesy of DPDx) www.cdc.gov/parasites/(https://www.cdc.gov/parasites/).

2.6. Prevention

Prevention implies taking measures at different levels, both in breeding and surveillance systems, as well as in the personal hygiene habits of people who consume pork. Some measures can be used to reduce the risk of infection for the consumption of infected meat in rural communities where pigs are maintained in backyard systems [18, 90, 91]:

- *In the backyard system.* Keep pigs raised in barnyards made with local materials and that prevent the access of pigs to areas that could be contaminated with pathogens such as *Toxoplasma gondii*, *Taenia solium* and *Trichinella spiralis*. Avoid areas where pigs could be in contact with cats and mice. Do not implement the outdoor bathroom.
- *Personal habits.* Implement personal hygiene habits, such as washing hands with soap and water before eating, after going to the bathroom and after handling raw, meat as well as washing hands after handling pets, such as like cats.
- *Food preparation.* Cookpork meat at a temperature of 71°C before consumption and avoid ingesting half-cooked meat; wash and disinfect raw fruits and vegetables and consume UV-treated water or boil and wash all kitchen utensils that have had contact with raw meat. Keep food out of reach of cats, and avoid the consumption of meat and organs such as the tongue and viscera that have visible nodules.
- *Personal health.* Deworm twice a year. All members of the family must be dewormed.

With simple actions implemented in communities with backyard systems, the risk of infection can be greatly reduced, and this ensures that backyard systems are a safe source of protein for people.

3. ABOUT OUR RESEARCH

In our experience, we carried out studies of *T. gondii* in samples of serum and tissue from pigs in southeastern Mexico. We will describe the methodologies of *T. gondii* detection that we carried out in our laboratory.

3.1. Determination of Anti-Igg Antibodies against *T. Gondii* through an Enzyme-Linked Immunosorbent Assay (ELISA)

Blood samples from the cava vein (Vacutainer tubes without anticoagulant) of pigs were collected at slaughter, and the samples were kept in refrigerated until they reached the laboratory. To obtain the serum, the samples were centrifuged for 10 min at 448 g. The serum samples were individually labeled and stored at -20°C until they were processed. The presence of IgG specific antibodies against *T. gondii* was determined using an indirect ELISA test (Human-GmbH, Wiesbaden, GER). The technique has been adapted according to Figueroa-Castillo [92] using a secondary antibody, anti-swine IgG-HRP (Catalog no. J3007, Santa Cruz, Inc., CA). The serum samples were evaluated at a concentration of 1:100, and IgG secondary antibodies were used at a dilution of 1:5000 [48]. A commercial normal swine serum (Catalog no. B2613; Santa Cruz, Inc., CA) was used as a negative control, and a serum from pigs previously tested by nested PCR (nPCR) as positive (in tissue sample), and an ELISA seropositive was used as the positive control. The optical density was measured at 450 nm using a spectrophotometer (xMark, Bio-Rad). The cutoff point was the average of the negative control plus three standard deviations.

3.2. Molecular Test

3.2.1. DNA Extraction from Pork Samples

DNA from tissue samples was predigested in pepsin solution, which was previously described (Table 4) [93]. Then, the protocol of the commercial kit, DNeasy Blood and Tissue (QIAGEN GmbH, Hilden, Germany), was followed. To assess the absence of endogenous inhibitors for PCR amplification, a housekeeping gene, glyceraldehyde 3-phosphate dehydrogenase (GAPDH) was analyzed in each DNA sample with real-time PCR [94].

Table 4. Materials used for isolation of DNA in pork samples in the southeast of Mexico

Sample	Materials and methods
Isolation of DNA in pork samples (50 grs)	Predigestion whit acid pepsin solution [93]* *Acid pepsin solution (Pepsin 2.6 g; NaC1, 5.0 g; HCI 7.0 mL and distilled water to make 500 ml, pH ~ 1.10-1.20). Phosphate buffered saline (PBS, pH 7.2) Sodium bicarbonate (pH ~ 8.3) Saline solution Blender Plastic jar Layers of gauze Plastic pipettes Follow the protocol for Tissue samples of DNeasy Blood and Tissue Kit (QIAGEN)
General consumables	Pipets and filter tips Vortex Microcentrifuge tubes (1.5mL) Microcentrifuge Centrifuge Thermomixer for heating at 56°C Reagents of DNeasy Blood and Tissue Kit (QIAGEN) Ethanol (96-100%)

3.2.2. Protocol for the Detection of T. gondii DNA in Pork Samples through a Nested Polymerase Chain Reaction (nPCR)

After the DNA extraction step, nPCR was performed to amplify a fragment of 390 bp of the SAG1 gene (encoding the main surface protein of *T. gondii*) [81], using a 96-well Veriti thermocycler (Applied Biosystems). The primers used were external forward 5'-GTTCTAACCACGC ACCCTGAG-3' and external reverse 5'- AAGAGTGGGAGGCTCT GTGA-3'. In the second amplification, the internal primers used were inner forward 5'-CAATGTGCACCTGTAGGAAGC-3' and inner reverse 5'-GTGGT TCTCCGTCGGTGTGAG-3'. The first amplification conditions were as follows: 1X Colorless GoTaq Flexi Buffer (PROMEGA); 2mM $MgCl_2$; 0.8 mm dNTPs; 0.5 μM for both the forward and reverse primers; 1.5 U Taq polymerase (GoTaq Flexi DNA Polymerase); and a 2 μL DNA sample in a final volume of 25 µL. The second amplification conditions had the same conditions as the first PCR, except that in this case, the concentration used for the forward and reverse primers was modified to 0.3 µM and as a template for the second round, 2 µL of the product was used from the first round of PCR. The nPCR conditions in the first run were 95°C for 5 min, followed by 30 cycles of 94°C for 30 s, 55°C for 1 min, and 72°C for 2 min. In the second run, the conditions were 95°C for 5 min, followed by 35 cycles of 94°C for 30 s, 60°C for 1 min, and 72°C for 1.5 min. The DNA from *T. gondii* axenic tachyzoite culture was used as a positive control, and a reaction without DNA was used as a negative control in each round of nPCR. The amplification products were observed on 1.5% agarose gel stained with ethidium bromide (10 mg/mL in H_2O).

3.2.3. Protocol for Detection of T. gondii DNA in Pork Samples through a Real Time Quantitative Polymerase Chain Reaction (qPCR)

The primers and Taqman probe amplified a fragment of 62 bp of the B1 gene of *T. gondii*, and the conditions have been previously described [95]. The specific primers used are GENE B1 TG-TX2F (5'-CTAGTATCGTGCGGCAATGTG-3') and GENE B1 TG-TX2R (5'-GGCAGCGTCTCTTCCTCTTTT-3') and a TaqMan probe (5'-(6-FAM)-CCACCTCGCCTCTTGG-(NFQ-MGB)-3'). Each qPCR reactionwas carried out in a final volume of 25 µL. The reaction conditions were as follow: 1X TaqMan Universal PCR Master Mix (PE Applied Biosystems) at an adjusted $MgCl_2$ concentration of 5 mM, 0.90 µM of each primer, 0.25 µL of the marker probe and 100 ng of purified DNA from the tissue. The amplification conditions were the following: initial incubation for 2 min at 50°C, followed by 10 min at 95°C, followed by 40 cycles of 95°C for 15 s and 60°C for 1 min. For the absolute quantification of the parasites, serial dilutions (from 1×10^{-2} to 1×10^5 parasites/mL) were performed by duplicated with known amounts of parasites/mL (tachyzoites) to construct the standard curves for *T. gondii* quantification. The parasite load determinations were performed by a linear regression analysis of the Ct values from known amounts of protozoan DNA to determine the *T. gondii* cell equivalents. The parasite load found in each tissue (estimated as a function of the Ct relative position from each sample with the Ct of the standard curve values) was divided per g of the sample to obtain the parasites/g by tissue. The results were expressed as *T. gondii* – equivalents (1 parasite equivalent = 68 femtograms of *T. gondii* DNA).

CONCLUSION

The human population is increasing every day and with it the demand for food of animal origin. Despite the fact that the implementation of intensive systems in the raising of pigs has drastically reduced the prevalence of *T. solium, T. gondii* and *T. spiralis* in developed countries, in rural regions of Mexico, it is still common to raise animals in backyard systems. Backyard farming systems are characterized by unhealthy conditions, a lack of confinement facilities, animals with poor diet, and inadequate health care. In addition, these animals are commonly slaughtered in the same homes where they are raised; therefore the rigorous inspection processes for the search of the cysts in their tissues are not carried out with cysts passing from their meat directly to the local consumers. This represents a high risk of infection for the population if this meat is consumed raw or undercooked.

In Mexico, studies of these three parasites *T. solium, T. gondii* and *T. spiralis*, in pigs are scarce dated, which makes it difficult to know the current epidemiological status of these agents. Moreover, it is alarming that in the country there are still outbreaks of cysticercosis/taeniasis, toxoplasmosis and trichinosis in the human population, which could indicate that the presence of these parasites in pigs for consumption is being underestimated. The data found in the literature show that these three agents in pork have a high impact on the health of the population; however, their detection is not mandatory. Unfortunately, the raising of backyard pigs is the key to the maintenance of these zoonoses. In addition, until measures are taken to improve production systems, the cycle of *T. solium, T. gondii* and *T. spiralis* will continue in the food chain. On the other hand, the breeding tendencies of animals in friendly conditions, free from stress and grazing, have made

Pork Foodborne Parasites of Public Health Interest in Mexico 67

this parasite reemerge due to the greater exposure of pigs to the contaminated environments.

Prevention measures should be taken when cooking pork carcasses at optimal temperatures (71°C or 160°F) to inactivate the tissue cysts of *T. solium, T. gondii* and *T. spiralis* and thus avoid the risk of infection. Other measures for the prevention of these diseases can be contribute to reducing outbreaks in Mexico by increasing the infrastructure in health services in marginalized communities, the implementation of dissemination campaigns regarding the epidemiology of these diseases among communities, and fostering habits of personal hygiene and good practices in breeding of pigs in backyard systems.

REFERENCES

[1] Djurković-Djaković, O., Bobić, B., Nikolić, A., Klun, I., Dupouy-Camet, J. (2013). Pork as a source of human parasitic infection. *Clin Microbiol Infect,* 19: 586-594.

[2] Boireau, P., Vallée, I., Gajadhar, A. A., Wang, X., Mingyuan, L. (2015). The role of regulatory and standard-setting organizations in the control of neglected foodborne parasites In A. A. Gajadhar (Ed), *Foodborne Parasites in the Food Supply Web.* Woodhead Publishing (pp. 429-444)

[3] Davies, P. R. (2010). Pork Safety: Achievements and Challenges. *Zoonoses Public Health,* 57: 1–5.

[4] Torgerson, P. R., Devleesschauwer, B., Praet, N., Speybroeck, N., Willingham, A. L., et al. (2015). World Health Organization Estimates of the Global and Regional Disease Burden of 11 Foodborne Parasitic Diseases, 2010: A Data Synthesis. *PLoS Med,* 12(12): e1001920.

[5] Davies, P. R. (2011). Intensive swine production and pork safety. *Foodborne Pathog Dis,* 8: 189-201.

[6] Food and Agriculture Organization of the United Nations/World Organization for Animal Health/World Bank. (2010). Good practices for biosecurity in the pig sector – Issues and options in developing and

transition countries. *FAO Animal Production and Health Paper No. 169.* Rome, FAO. Available at: http://www.fao.org/3/a-i1435e.pdf.

[7] Gamble H. R. (2015). Trends in Food Production Practices Relative to Foodborne Parasites. In A. A. Gajadhar (Ed), *Foodborne Parasites in the Food Supply Web: Occurrence and Control.* Woodhead Publishing (Pp. 11-21).

[8] Gajadhar A. A. (2015). Introduction to foodborne parasites In A. A. Gajadhar (Ed), *Foodborne Parasites in the Food Supply Web: Occurrence and Control.* Woodhead Publishing (Pp. 3-9).

[9] Secretary of Agriculture, Livestock, Rural Development, Fisheries and Food (SAGARPA). (2016). Agreement by means of which the Diseases and Exotic and Endemic Pests of Obligatory Notification of Terrestrial and Aquatic Animals are Made Known in the Mexican States. *Official Journal of the Federation.* Available at: https://www.gob.mx/cms/uploads/attachment/file/210722/ACUERDOmediante_el _cual_se_dan_a_conocer_en_los_Estados_Unidos_Mexicanos_las_e nfermedades_y_plagas_exoticas_y_endemicas_de_notificacion_oblig atoria_de_los_animales_terrestres_y_acuaticos.pdf.

[10] Medina, L. M. S. Ramírez, A. A. Pérez, T. E. Pacheco, G. C. Ruvalcaba, B. S. et al. (2007). Viability of *Trichinella spiralis* in Meat Pig on Various Experimental Conditions of Conservation. *Memories of IX of the Congress of Food Science and the V Forum on Food Science and Technology* (Pp. 235-243).

[11] Secretary of Agriculture, Livestock, Rural Development, Fisheries and Food (SAGARPA). 2018. *Directorate of Establishments Type Federal Inspection.* Available at: https://www.gob.mx/cms/uploads/attach ment/file/399844/Directorio_General_12-10-2018.pdf

[12] Cruz-Licea, V., Plancarte-Crespo, A., Morán-Álvarez, I. C. (2003). Teniosis and Cysticercosis in food traders in markets in an area of Mexico City. *Latin American Parasitol.* 58: 1-2.

[13] Jiménez-Cardoso, E., Caballero-García, M. L., Uribe-Gutiérrez, G., Trejo-Hernández, E., Gay-Jiménez. (2005). Frequency of *Trichinella spiralis* in blood and muscle of horses slaughtered in two different

slaughterhouses, one industrial and the other rural type in the State of Mexico, Mexico. *Vet Mex*, 36(3): 269-278.

[14] Zolfaghari Emameh, R., Purmonen, S., Sukura, A., Parkkila, S. (2017). Surveillance and diagnosis of zoonotic foodborne parasites. *Food Sci Nutr*, 6(1): 3-17.

[15] Center for Food Security and Public Health (CFSPH). (2005). Iowa State University. *Taenia infections*. Available at: http://www. cfsph.iastate.edu/Factsheets/pdfs/taenia.pdf.

[16] Pawlowski, Z. S. (2002). *Taenia solium*: Basic biology and transmission. In: Singh, G., Prabhakar, S. (Ed). *Taenia solium cysticercosis. From basic to clinical Science*. CABI Publishing. India. (Pp. 1-13).

[17] Chiodini, P. L., Moody, A. H., Manser, D. W. (2003). *Atlas of medical Helminthology and protozoology*. Fourth edition, Churchill-Livingstone. London. Pp. 82.

[18] Pan American Health Oraganization-World Health Organization (PAHO-WHO). (2003). *Zoonoses and communicable diseases common to man and animals*. Vol. III. Parasitoses. Third Edition. Washington, D.C. Pp. 404.

[19] O'Neal, S., Townes, J., Keene, B. (2015). *Taeniasis and Cysticercosis. Investigative guidelines*. Oregon Public Health Division. Available at: https://www.oregon.gov/oha/ph/diseasesconditions/communicabledis ease/reportingcommunicabledisease/reportingguidelines/Documents/t aeniasis_cyst_guideline.pdf.

[20] Rodriguez-Canul, R., Allan, J. C., Dominguez, J. L., Villegas, S., Cob, L., Rodriguez, R. I., et al. (1998). Application of an immunoassay to determine risk factors associated with porcine cysticercosis in rural areas of Yucatan, Mexico. *Vet Parasitol*, 79: 165-80.

[21] Rodriguez-Canul, R., Fraser, A., Allan, J. C., Dominguez-Alpizar, J. L., Argaez-Rodriguez, F., Craig, P. S. (1999). Epidemiological study of *Taenia solium* taeniasis/cysticercosis in a rural village in Yucatan State, Mexico. *Ann Trop Med Parasitol*, 93: 57-67.

[22] Widdowson, M. A., Cook, A. J., Williams, J. J., Argaes, F., Rodriguez, I., Dominguez, J. L., Rodriguez, R. (2000). Investigation of risk factors

for porcine *Taenia solium* cysticercosis: a multiple regression analysis of a cross-sectional study in the Yucatan Peninsula, Mexico. *Trans R Soc Trop Med Hyg,* 94(6): 620-624.

[23] Sarti-Gutierrez, E. J., Schantz, P. M., Lara-Aguilera, R., Gomez-Dandoy, H., Flisser, A. (1988). *Taenia solium* taeniasis and cysticercosis in a Mexican village. *Trop Med Parasitol,* 39(3): 194-198.

[24] Sarti, E., Schantz, P. M., Plancarte, A., Wilson, M., Gutierrez, I. O., Lopez, A. S., et al. (1992a). Prevalence and Risk Factors for *Taenia Solium* Taeniasis and Cysticercosis in Humans and Pigs in a Village in Morelos, Mexico. *Ame J Trop Med Hygiene.* 46: 677-685.

[25] Sarti, E., Flisser, A., Schantz, P. M., Gleizer, M., Loya, M., Plancarte, A., et al. (1997). Development and evaluation of a health education intervention against *Taenia solium* in a rural community in Mexico. *Am J Trop Med Hyg,* 56(2): 127-132.

[26] Morales, J., Martínez, J. J., Rosetti, M., Fleury, A., Maza, V., Hernandez, M., et al. (2008). Spatial distribution of *Taenia solium* porcine cysticercosis within a rural area of Mexico. *PLoS Negl Trop Dis,* 2(9):e284.

[27] Morales, J., Martínez, J. J., Villalobos, N., Hernández, M., Ramírez, R., Salgado-Estrada, B., et al. (2018). Persistent *Taenia solium* Cysticercosis in the State of Morelos, Mexico: Human and Porcine Seroprevalence. *J Parasitol,* 104(5): 465-472.

[28] Sarti-G, E., Schantz, P. M., Aguilera, J., Lopez, A. (1992b). Epidemiologic observations on porcine cysticercosis in a rural community of Michoacan State, Mexico. *Vet parasitol,* 41:195-201.

[29] de Aluja, A. S., Suárez-Marín, R., Sciutto-Conde, E., Morales-Soto, J., Martínez-Maya, J. J., Villalobos, N. (2014). Evaluation of the impact of a control program against Taeniasis-Cysticercosis (*Taenia solium*). *Sal Pub Mex.* 56(3): 259-265.

[30] Aluja-Schunemann, A., Scuitto-Conde, E., Suárez-Marín, C., Pérez-Gómez, J. G., Celis-Trejo, A. J., López-Rodríguez, A., et al. (2013). A programme to control taeniosis-cysticercosis (*Taenia solium*) in

Mexico collaboration agreement SENASICA-UNAM. *Vet Electronic Magazine*, 14(11B): 1-17.

[31] Altagracia-Martínez, M., Kravzov-Jinich, J., Moreno-Bonett, C., López-Naranjo, F., Martínez-Núñez, J. M. (2012). The neglected diseases of Latin America and the Caribbean: a problem for public global health. *Mex J Pharmaceutical Scie,* 43: 33-41.

[32] Secretaria de Salud (SSA). (2018). *Epidemiological Bulletin. National Epidemiological Surveillance System. Mexico.* Available at: https://www.gob.mx/cms/uploads/attachment/file/406832/sem42.pdf.

[33] Severance, E. G., Xiao, J., Jones-Brando, L., Sabunciyan, S., Li, Y., Pletnikov, M., et al. (2016). *Toxoplasma gondii.* A Gastrointestinal Pathogen Associated with Human Brain Diseases. *Int Rev of Neurobiol*, 131: 143-163

[34] Tenter, A. M., Heckeroth, A. R., Weiss, L. M. (2000). *Toxoplasma gondii*: from animals to humans. *Int J Parasitol,* 30: 1217–1258.

[35] Belluco, S., Mancin, M., Conficoni, D., Simonato, G., Pietrobelli, M., Ricci, A. (2016). Investigating the Determinants of *Toxoplasma gondii* Prevalence in Meat: A Systematic Review and Meta-Regression. *PLoS ONE*, 11(4): e0153856.

[36] Bosch-Driessen, L. E., Berendschot, T. T., Ongkosuwito, J. V., Rothova, A. (2002). Ocular toxoplasmosis: clinical features and prognosis of 154 patients. *Ophthalmology.* 109: 869–878.

[37] Kimball, A. C., Kean, B. H., Fuchs, F. (1974). Toxoplasmosis: Risk variations in New York City obstetric patients. *Am J Obst Gynecol,* 119: 208–214.

[38] Dubey J. P, and Beattie, C. P. (1988). *Toxoplasmosis of animals and man.* CRC Press, Boca Raton, Florida, 220 p.

[39] Cook, A. J., Gilbert, R. E., Buffolano, W., Zufferey, J., Petersen, E., Jenum, P. A., et al. (2000). Sources of toxoplasma infection in pregnant women: European multicentre case-control study. European Research Network on Congenital Toxoplasmosis. *BMJ,* 321: 142–147.

[40] Hill D. E., Dubey J. P. (2018). *Toxoplasma gondii*. In: Ortega Y. R., Sterling C. R. (eds) *Foodborne Parasites. Food Microbiology and Food Safety.* Springer International Publishing. (Pp. 119-138).

[41] Dubey, J. P., Murrell, K. D., Fayer, R., & Schad, G. A. (1986). Distribution of *Toxoplasma gondii* tissue cysts in commercial cuts of pork. *J Am Vet Med Assoc*, 188: 1035–1037.

[42] Dubey, J. P., Lunney, J. K., Shen, S. K., Kwok, O. C., Ashford, D. A., Thulliez, P. (1996). Infectivity of low numbers of *Toxoplasma gondii* oocysts to pigs. *J Parasitol*, 82: 438-443.

[43] Alvarado-Esquivel, C., García-Machado, C., Alvarado-Esquivel, D., González-Salazar, A. M., Briones-Fraire, C., Vitela-Corrales, J., et al. (2011). Seroprevalence of *Toxoplasma gondii* infection in domestic pigs in Durango State, Mexico. *J Parasitol*, 97(4): 616-619.

[44] Alvarado-Esquivel, C., Vazquez-Morales, R. F., Colado-Romero, E. E., Guzmán-Sánchez, R., Liesenfeld, O., Dubey, J. P. (2015). Prevalence of infection with *Toxoplasma gondii* in landrace and mixed breed pigs slaughtered in Baja California Sur State, Mexico. *Eur J Microbiol Immunol*, 5(1): 112-115.

[45] García-Vázquez, Z., Rosario-Crus, R., Diaz-Garcia, G., Hernandez-Baumgarten, O. (1993). Seroprevalence of *Toxoplasma gondii* infection in cattle, swine and goats in four Mexican states. *Preventive Veterinary Medicine*, 17; 127-132.

[46] Galván-Ramirez, M. L., Madriz-Elisondo, A. L., Rico-Torres, C. P., Luna-Pastén, H., Rodríguez-Pérez, L. R., Rincón-Sánchez, A. R., et al. (2010). Frequency of *Toxoplasma gondii* in pork meat in Ocotlán, Jalisco, Mexico. *J Food Prot*, 73(6): 1121-1123.

[47] Alvarado-Esquivel, C., Romero-Salas, D., García-Vázquez, Z., Crivelli-Diaz, M., Barrientos-Morales, M., Lopez-de-Buen, L., Dubey, J. P. (2014). Seroprevalence and correlates of *Toxoplasma gondii* infection in domestic pigs in Veracruz State, Mexico. *Trop Anim Health Prod*, 46(4): 705-709.

[48] Ortega-Pacheco, A., Acosta-Viana, K. Y., Guzman-Marin, E., Uitzil-Álvarez, B., Rodríguez-Buenfil, J. C., Jimenez-Coello, M. (2011). Infection dynamic of *Toxoplasma gondii* in two fattening pig farms exposed to high and low cat density in an endemic region. *Vet Parasitol*, 175(3-4):367-371.

Pork Foodborne Parasites of Public Health Interest in Mexico 73

[49] Ortega-Pacheco, A., Acosta-Viana, K. Y., Guzmán-Marín, E., Segura-Correa, J. C., Álvarez-Fleites, M., Jiménez-Coello, M. (2013). Prevalence and Risk Factors of *Toxoplasma gondii* in Fattening Pigs Farm from Yucatan, Mexico. *Biomed Res Int.* 2013: 231497.

[50] Jimenez-Coello, M., Acosta-Viana, K. Y., Guzman-Marin, E., Gutierrez-Ruiz, E. J., Rodriguez-Vivas, R. I., Bolio-González, M. E., Ortega-Pacheco, A. (2013). The occurrence of *Toxoplasma gondii* antibodies in backyard pigs and cats from an endemic tropical area of Mexico. *Trop Subtrop Agroecosys*, 16: 89-92.

[51] Hernández-Cortazar, I. B., Acosta-Viana, K. Y., Guzmán-Marin, E., Ortega-Pacheco, A., Torres-Acosta, J. F., Jimenez-Coello, M. (2016). Presence of *Toxoplasma gondii* in Pork Intended for Human Consumption in Tropical Southern Mexico. *Foodborne Pathog Dis,* 13(12): 695-699.

[52] Dzib-Paredes, G. F., Rosado-Aguilar, J. A., Acosta-Viana, K. Y., Ortega-Pacheco, A., Hernández-Cortazar, I. B., Guzman-Marin, E., Jiménez-Coello, M. (2016). Seroprevalence and parasite load of *Toxoplasma gondii* in Mexican hairless pig (Sus scrofa) tissues from the Southeast of Mexico. *Vet Parasitol,* 229: 45-49.

[53] Alvarado-Esquivel, C., Estrada-Malacón, M. A., Reyes-Hernández, S. O., Pérez-Ramírez, J. A., Trujillo-López, J. I., Villena, I., Dubey, J. P. (2012). High prevalence of *Toxoplasma gondii* antibodies in domestic pigs in Oaxaca State, Mexico. *J Parasitol,* 98(6): 1248-1250.

[54] Hernandez-Cortazar, I., Acosta-Viana, K. Y., Ortega-Pacheco, A., Guzman-Marin, E., Aguilar-Caballero, A. J., Jiménez-Coello, M. (2015). Toxoplasmosis in Mexico: epidemiological situation in humans and animals. *Rev Inst Med Trop Sao Paulo*, 57(2): 93-103.

[55] Dupouy-Camet, J. (2000). Trichinellosis: a worldwide zoonosis. *Vet Parasitol,* 93: 191-200.

[56] Messiaen, P., Forier, A., Vanderschueren, S., Theunissen, C., Nijs, J., Van Esbroeck, M., et al. (2016). Outbreak of Trichinellosis related to eating imported wild boar meat, Belgium. *Euro Surveill,* 21(37): 30341.

74 I.B. Hernandez-Cortazar, E. Guzman-Marin, K.Y. Acosta-Viana et al.

[57] Capo, V., Despommier, D. (1996). Clinical aspects of infection with *Trichinella spp. Clin. Microbiol. Rev.* 9: 47–54.

[58] Ancelle, T. (1998). History of Trichinellosis outbreaks linked to horsemeat consumption 1975–1998. *Euro surveill,* 3, 86–89.

[59] Pozio, E., Murrell, K. D. (2006). Systematics and epidemiology of Trichinella. *Adv Parasitol.* 63: 367–439.

[60] Ortega-Pierres, M. G., Arriaga, C., Yépez-Mulia, L. (2000). Epidemiology of trichinellosis in Mexico, Central and South America. *Vet Parasitol,* 93(3-4): 201-225.

[61] Sun, G. G., Song, Y. Y., Jiang, P., Ren, H. N., Yan, S. W., Han, Y., et al. (2018). Characterization of a *Trichinella spiralis* putative serine protease. Study of its potential as sero-diagnostic tool. *PLoS Negl Trop Dis,* 12(5): e0006485.

[62] Murrell, D., Pozio, E. (2011). Worldwide occurrence and impact of human Trichinellosis, 1986–2009. *Emer Infect Dis*, 12: 2194-2202.

[63] Murrell, K. D. 2016. The dynamics of *Trichinella spiralis* epidemiology: Out to pasture?. *Vet Parasitol,* 231: 92-96.

[64] Vázquez-Tsuji, O., Campos-Rivera, T. (2012). Epidemiology of Trichinosis in Mexico. *J Infect Dis Pediatrics*, 26: 166-167.

[65] Tay Zavala, J., Sánchez Vega, J., Ruiz Sánchez, D., Calderón Romero, L., García Yañez, Y., Alonso, T., et al. (2004). Current Status of our knowledge about Trichinellosis in the Mexican Republic, report of new infected localities. *Rev Fac Med UNAM,* 47: 96-100.

[66] Reveles-Hernández, R. G., Saldivar-Elías, S. J., Maldonado-Tapia, C., Muñoz-Escobedo, J. J., Moreno-García, M. A. (2011). Evaluation of the infection of *Trichinella spiralis* in gonadectomized pigs, Zacatecas, Mexico. *Peruvian Medical Act*, 28(4): 211-216.

[67] Chávez-Guajardo, E., Muñoz-Escobedo, J. J., Reveles-Hernández, G., Rivas-Gutierréz, J., Moreno-García, A. (2007). Effect of temperature on the viability and infectivity of *T. spiralis. AVFT*, 26 (2): 1-5.

[68] Arriaga, C., Muriz, E., Morilla, A., Ortega-Pierrest, G. (1989). *Trichinella spiralis*: Recognition of Muscle Larva Antigens during Experimental Infection of Swine and Its Potential Use in Diagnosis. *Exp parasitol.* 69: 363-372.

Pork Foodborne Parasites of Public Health Interest in Mexico 75

[69] Martínez-Barbabosa, I., Vázquez-Tsuji, O., Romero-Cabello, R., Gutiérrez-Quiroz, M., García-Yáñez, Y., Fernández-Presas, A. M., Campos-Rivera, T. (2001). Search for *Trichinella spiralis* in pork that is sold in butcher shops of the Federal District. *Vet Mex*, 31.

[70] Monroy, H., Flores-Trujillo, M., Benitez, E., Arriaga, C. (2001). Swine trichinellosis in slaughterhouses of the metropolitan area of Toluca. *Parasite*, 8: S249-S251

[71] Gonzalez, A. E., Cama, V., Gilman, R. H., Tsang, V. C., Pilcher, J. B., Chavera, A., et al. (1990). Prevalence and comparation of serological assays, necropsy and tongue examination for the diagnosis of porcine cisticercosis in Peru. *Am J Trop Med Hyg,* 43, 194-199.

[72] Davelois, K., Escalante, H., Jara, C. (2016). Western Blot diagnostic yield for simultaneous antibody-detection in patients with human cysticercosis, hydatidosis, and human fascioliasis. *Rev Peru Med Exp Public Health*, 33(4): 616-624.

[73] Sciutto, E., Martínez, J. J., Villalobos, N. M., Hernández, M., José M. V., Beltrán, C., et al. (1998). Limitations of current diagnostic procedures for the diagnosis of *Taenia solium* cysticercosis in rural pigs. *Vet Parasitol,* 79, 299-313.

[74] Herrera-García, S.C., de Aluja, A. S., Méndez-Aguilar. (2007). Use of ultrasound to diagnose porcine cysticersosis. *Vet Mex*, 30, 125-133.

[75] Al-Adhami, B. H., Gajadhar, A. A. 2014. A new multi-host species indirect ELISA using protein A/G conjugate for detection of anti-Toxoplasma gondii IgG antibodies with comparison to ELISA-IgG, agglutination assay and Western blot. *Vet Parasitol* 200, 66-73.

[76] Villard, O., Cimon, B., L'Ollivier, C., Fricker-Hidalgo, H., Godineau, N., Houze, S., et al. (2016). Serological diagnosis of *Toxoplasma gondii* infection: Recommendations from the French National Reference Center for Toxoplasmosis. *Diagn Microbiol Infect Dis.* 84(1): 22-33.

[77] Feitosa, T. F., Ribeiro-Vilela, V. L., de Almeida-Neto, J. L., Dos-Santos, A., de-Morais, D. F., Alves, B. F., et al. (2017). High genetic diversity in *Toxoplasma gondii* isolates from pigs at slaughterhouses

in Paraíba state, northeastern Brazil: Circulation of new genotypes and Brazilian clonal lineages. *Vet Parasitol*, 244, 76-80.

[78] Steinparzer, R., Reisp, K., Grunberger, B., Kofer, J., Schmoll, F., Sattler, T. (2014). Comparison of different commercial serological tests for the detection of *Toxoplasma gondii* antibodies in serum of naturally exposed pigs. *Zoonoses Public Health*, 15, 1–6.

[79] Forbes, L. B., Parker, S. E., Gajadhar, A. A. 2012. Performance of commercial ELISA and agglutination test kits for the detection of anti-*Toxoplasma gondii* antibodies in serum and muscle fluid of swine infected with 100, 300, 500 or 1000 oocysts. *Vet Parasitol*. 190, 362-367.

[80] Gazzonis, A. L., Marangi, M., Villa, L., Ragona, M. E., Olivieri, E., Zanzani, S. A., et al. (2018). *Toxoplasma gondii* infection and biosecurity levels in fattening pigs and sows: serological and molecular epidemiology in the intensive pig industry (Lombardy, Northern Italy). *Parasitol Res*, 117, 539-546.

[81] Su C, Shwab EK, Zhou P, et al. (2010). Moving towards an integrated approach to molecular detection and identification of *Toxoplasma gondii*. *Parasitol,* 137: 1–11.

[82] Opsteegh, M., Langelaar, M., Sprong, H., Hartog, L.D., De Craeye, S., Bokken, G., et al. (2010). Direct detection and genotyping of *Toxoplasma gondii* in meat samples using magnetic capture and PCR. *Int J Food Microbiol*, 139, 193-201.

[83] Gisbert-Algaba, I., Geerts, M., Jennes, M., Coucke, W., Opsteegh, M., Cox, E., et al. (2017). A more sensitive, efficient and ISO 17025 validated Magnetic Capture real time PCR method for the detection of archetypal *Toxoplasma gondii* strains in meat. *Int J Parasitol,* 47, 875-884.

[84] Forbes, L. B., Parker, S., Scandrett, W. B. (2003). Comparison of a modified digestion assay with trichinoscopy for the detection of Trichinella larvae in pork. *J Food Prot*. 66(6): 1043-6.

[85] Konecsni, K., Scheller, C., Scandrett, B., Buholzer, Gajadhar, A. (2017). Evaluation of the PrioCHECK™ Trichinella AAD Kit for the

digestion and recovery of larvae in pork, horse meat and wild meat. *Vet Parasitol*, 243: 267-271.

[86] Bokken, G. C., Bergwerff, A. A., van Knapen, F. (2012). A novel bead-based assay to detect specific antibody responses against *Toxoplasma gondii* and *Trichinella spiralis* simultaneously in sera of experimentally infected swine. *BMC Vet Res.* 8, 36.

[87] Fu, B. Q., Li, W. H., Gai, W. Y., Yao, J. X., Qu, Z. Q., Xie, Z. Z., et al. (2013). Detection of anti-Trichinella antibodies in serum of experimentally-infected swine by immunochromatographic strip. *Vet Parasitol*, 194: 125-127.

[88] Cuttell, L., Corley, S. W., Gray, C. P., Vanderlinde, P. B., Jackson L. A., Traub, R. J. (2012). Real-time PCR as a surveillance tool for the detection of Trichinella infection in muscle samples from wildlife. *Vet Parasitol*, 188: 285-293.

[89] Lin, Z., Cao, J., Zhang, H., Zhou, Y., Deng, M., Li, G., Zhou, J. (2013). Comparison of three molecular detection methods for detection of Trichinella in infected pigs. *Parasitol Res*, 112: 2087-2093.

[90] United States Department of Agriculture (USDA). (2011). *Parasites and Foodborne Illness.* Food Safety and Inspection Service. Available at: https://www.fsis.usda.gov/wps/wcm/connect/48a0685a-61ce-4235-b2d7-f07f53a0c7c8/Parasites_and_Foodborne_Illness.pdf?MOD=AJPERES.

[91] Djurkovic-Djakovic, O., Bobic, B., Nokolic, A., Klun, I., Dupouy-Camet, J., (2013). Pork as source of human parasitic infection. *Clin Microbiol Infect*, 19: 586-594.

[92] Figueroa-Castillo, J. A., Duarte-Rosas, V., Juárez-Acevedo, M., Luna-Pastén, H., Correa, D., (2006). Prevalence of *Toxoplasma gondii* antibodies in rabbits (Orytogalus cuniculus) from Mexico. *J. Parasitol*, 92(2): 394–395.

[93] Dubey, J. P. (1998). Refinement of pepsin digestion method for isolation of *Toxoplasma gondii* from infected tissues. *Vet Parasitol*, 74: 75-77.

[94] Cencig, S., Coltel, N., Truyens, C., Carlier, Y., 2011. Parasitic loads in tissues of miceinfected with *Trypanosoma cruzi* and treated with AmBisome. *PLoS Negl. Trop. Dis.* 5 (6), e1216.

[95] Kompalic-Cristo, A., Frotta, C., Suárez-Mutis, M., Fernandes, O., Britto, C. (2007). Evaluation of a real-time PCR assay based on the repetitive B1 gene for the detection of *Toxoplasma gondii* in human peripheral blood. *Parasitol. Res,* 101: 619–625.

In: Pork Consumption and Health
Editor: Frank L. Moore
ISBN: 978-1-53614-991-3
© 2019 Nova Science Publishers, Inc.

Chapter 3

PORK MEAT CONSUMPTION AND SALMONELLOSIS INCIDENCE IN EUROPEAN COUNTRIES: AN ECOLOGIC STUDY

Alberto Arnedo-Pena[1], PhD and M. Rosario Pac-Sa[2], MD
[1]Department of Health Sciences,
Public University of Navarra, Pamplona, Spain
[2]International Health, Sub-delegation of Spain Government,
Castellon, Spain

ABSTRACT

Introduction: In European countries salmonellosis incidence is elevated and it is generally associated with the consumption of eggs, eggs-products and poultry meat, while *S.* Enteritidis is the more reported serotype. However, the incidence of *S* Typhimurium salmonellosis with its monophasic variant is increasing, and swine is considered as an important reservoir of *S.* Typhimurium. Our hypothesis is that pork meat consumption in European countries may be associated with salmonellosis incidence.

Material and methods: The average salmonellosis incidence rate in 31 European countries during the period 2013-2014 was obtained from European Centre for Disease Prevention and Control and European Food Safety Authority. Consumption of pork meat, bovine meat, poultry and eggs in these countries during 2013 was retrieved from the Food and Agriculture Organization. Socioeconomic, demographic, health organization and climate variables were taken from different sources in order to adjust the statistical models. First, Spearman's correlation coefficient was used to study the relationship salmonellosis and explanatory variables. Second, a multilevel linear regression analysis was carried out with two levels: region, occidental and oriental, European countries, and climate (Mediterranean, Atlantic, continental, and sub-arctic). Stata ®14 version was used in the statistical analysis.

Results: In the period, the average of salmonellosis incidence rate was 19.1 cases per 100,000 inhabitants (range 2.05-109.6), and the median of pork meat consumption was 34.96 kg/capita/year (range 21.01-52.56). In the multilevel model, salmonellosis incidence increases by 0.79 (95% CI [confidence interval] 0.11-1.48; p = 0.023) with the increase in pork meat consumption, adjusted by GINI index, -2.75 (95% CI -4.20- -1.30; p = 0.000). Egg consumption had no significant association with salmonellosis, (1.69 95% CI -0.70-4.07 p = 0.165). In addition a dose-response pork meat consumption and salmonellosis was found (p = 0.001). The interclass correlation coefficient was 0.31 (95% CI 0.04-0.83), the proportion of total salmonellosis variance among countries. The models presented acceptable goodness of fit tests. Limitations of this study include its ecological approach, national differences in salmonellosis report and control, no distinction of *Salmonella* outbreaks, and no differentiation among *Salmonella* serotypes.

Conclusion: Our study suggests that pork meat consumption is associated with salmonellosis incidence in European countries. An increment and optimization of control and prevention measures in the farm-to-consumption chain for pork products are recommended.

Keywords: *Salmonella, S.* Typhimurium, salmonellosis, foodborne diseases, pork, swine.

INTRODUCTION

Salmonellosis is a zoonosis with many animal species affected, including a wide variety of reservoirs of *Salmonella* bacteria which can infect human population by ingestion and contact. In general, consumption of animal products with *Salmonella* represents the principal mechanism of transmission (Silva et al. 2014).

Since the 1990s, thousands of salmonellosis cases have been reported each year in European countries. These infections were predominantly caused by *S.* Enteritidis; eggs, eggs-products, and poultry meat were their habitual vehicles (Dominguez et al. 2007). In 2016, *S.* Enteritidis is still the most frequent salmonellosis serotype, and specific control measures in poultry farms reduced their incidence. However, in the last 5 years this incidence has been maintained stable; laying hens, broilers and broiler meat were mainly risk factors (EFSA 2017). From data of 2005-2009, mathematical models found laying hens as the first source of salmonellosis, and pigs as a second source (De Knegt et al. 2015).

However, in recent years other *Salmonella* serotypes, such as *S.* Typhimuriun with their monophasic variant 4,5,12:i:-, have increased both in salmonellosis foodborne outbreaks and in sporadic cases (Mughini-Gras et al. 2014, Andreoli et al. 2017). Swine is the most important *S.* Typhimurium reservoir, and pig farms are crucial places of *Salmonella* transmission (Foley et al. 2008, Parada et al. 2017). In addition, a public health danger of the monophasic variant, including virulence and antibiotic multi-resistance, has been pointed out in different studies (Bonardi 2017, EFSA 2010). In contrast to *S.* Enteritidis, salmonellosis by *S.* Tyhpimurium is frequently associated with the consumption of contaminated pig, poultry, and bovine meat (EFSA 2010), affecting mainly children and elderly people, and causing foodborne outbreaks difficult to detect by traditional surveillance methods (Alt et al. 2015, Arnedo-Pena et al. 2017). In some countries like China, *S.* Typhimurium is a more frequently agent of salmonellosis than *S.*Enteritidis, and pork products have a high prevalence of *Salmonella* (Yan et al. 2017). In a review of foodborne outbreaks related to meat products (Omer et al. 2018*), S.* Typhimurium was the serovar more frequently associated with pork products consumption, and raw-cured fermented sausages were the foods with more implication.

Therefore, our aim is to study the consumption of different foods related to potential risk of salmonellosis. Our hypothesis is that pork meat consumption in European countries may be associated with salmonellosis incidence.

MATERIAL AND METHODS

In order to test our hypothesis, a multilevel linear regression analysis was carried out. Salmonellosis incidence in 31 European countries was obtained from European Centre Disease Prevention and Control (ECDPC 2016) and European Food Safety Authority (EFSA 2015) as laboratory-confirmed cases. The average of salmonellosis incidence rates in 2013 and 2014 in European countries was the dependent variable. Explanatory variables (predictors and confusion variables) were obtained from different sources:

- Statistic data from the Food and Agriculture Organization (FAOSTAT), pork meat consumption in European countries as the Food Balance Sheets as pig meat food supply quantity by kg/capita/year in the 2013 from 31 European countries. This is the last year with the correspondent information. In addition, other explanatory variables were obtained, such as consumption of poultry meat, eggs, bovine meat, by kg/capita/year for the same year.
- Median temperatures, 1th (low), and 99th (high) temperatures percentiles from 2014 were obtained from the World Bank Group through their climate change knowledge portal,
- The European Commission. Socioeconomic and demographic variables were gathered from EUROSAT in 2014, including: GINI index as coefficient of equalized disposable income, gross domestic product (GDP), percent population under 5 years old, percent population under 15 years old, percent rural population less 5.000 inhabitants, percent towns and suburbs population minimum 5,000 inhabitants (urban cluster), and percent city (high-density cluster) minimum 50,000 inhabitants. In addition, we included statistic data

Pork Meat Consumption and Salmonellosis Incidence ...

of healthcare organization: physicians by 100,000 inhabitants, and healthcare expenditure (euros) in 2015.

In multilevel models, two levels were considered. The first level was a region, considering occidental and oriental, west and east Europa. Occidental Europe included Austria, Belgium, Cyprus, Denmark, Finland, France, Germany, Greece, Iceland, Italy, Luxembourg, Malta, the Netherlands, Norway, Portugal, Spain, Sweden, United Kingdom, Ireland, and Switzerland. Oriental Europe included Bulgaria, Croatia, Check Republic, Estonia, Hungry, Latvia, Lithuania, Poland, Romania, Slovakia, and Slovenia. It may represent the political division of European countries for several decades, and it could define some specific characteristics, such as socioeconomic development, cultural influences, or food habits. The second level was climate since salmonellosis has been associated with climate characteristics (Lake 2017). In general, salmonellosis incidence is more frequent during the summer season of the year (Kovats et al. 2004), especially for *S*. Enteriditis. However, regarding *S*. Typhimurium, its incidence is less marked for the season of year. The climate of European countries is very heterogeneous, and several countries like Spain, Germany, Sweden or Italy, have different climate zones. Following the Köppen-Geiger system of climate zones in Europe and the PVSITES Consortium (2016), four climate zones were considered (Mediterranean, continental, Atlantic, and subarctic). The distribution of countries by climate zones was the following:

- *Mediterranean*: Cyprus, Greece, Italy, Malta, Portugal, and Spain.
- *Continental*: Austria, Bulgaria, Croatia, Czech Republic, Hungry, Luxembourg, Poland, Romania, Slovakia, Slovenia, and Switzerland.
- *Atlantic*: Belgium, Denmark, France, Germany, the Netherlands, United Kingdom, and Ireland.
- *Subarctic*: Estonia, Finland, Iceland, Latvia, Lithuania, Norway, and Sweden.

Statistical Methods

Averages, medians, and ranges were used in order to describe variables characteristics. Salmonellosis incidence rate corresponds to the average of 2013-2014 years with the purpose of avoiding potential extreme data due to *Salmonella* foodborne outbreaks. Several statistical tests were used in a bivariate analysis, including Spearman rank`s correlations test, which allows to study the strength of the relationship between salmonellosis incidence rates and explanatory variables in order to select these variables for multilevel models (Smyth et al. 2013). In addition, a test of trend was carried out to estimate the effect dose-response between pork meat consumption and salmonellosis incidences.

Multilevel linear regression models with two levels, region, and climate, were implemented under the hypothesis of a normal distribution of the variables in this study. First, a bivariate multilevel approach was generated with salmonellosis incidence and all explanatory variables one by one. Second, in order to obtain parsimonious and well-fitting model, the next multilevel models included salmonellosis incidence as dependent variable, and explanatory variables those that (i) had with a Spearman rank's correlation coefficients ≥ 0.20 and (ii) an association with salmonellosis incidence with a $p \leq 0.20$, in order to obtain parsimonious and well-fitted models. The final multilevel model was generated with all explanatory variables significantly associated with salmonellosis incidence ($p < 0.05$). 95% confidence intervals (CI) of regression coefficients were calculated. The models presented acceptable goodness of fit tests, considering deviance, Akaike's and Bayesian information criteria. Stata® version 14 was used for all calculations.

RESULTS

Descriptive Approach

During 2013 and 2014, 90,576 new cases of salmonellosis were reported as an annual average in 31 European countries. Salmonellosis incidence rates, some food consumptions associated with salmonellosis and climate temperatures of these countries are presented in Table 1. The average salmonellosis incidence rate was 19.1 cases per 100,000 inhabitants, ranging a minimum 2.1 per 100,000 inhabitants in Portugal (214 cases) and a maximum 109.6 per 100,000 inhabitants in the Czech Republic (11,634 cases). In 2013, the median pork meat consumption was 34.96 kg/capita/year (range 21.01-52.56). Countries with the highest pork meat consumption were Austria 52.56 kg/capita/year, Germany 51.81 kg/capita/year, and Spain 48.92 kg/capita/year. Countries with the lowest pork meat consumption were Norway 21.01 kg/capita/year, Denmark 24.89 kg/capita/year, and Romania 25.3 kg/capita/year. The median of eggs, poultry and bovine meat consumptions were 12.2 kg/capita/year (range 7.53-16.05), 21.06 kg/capita/year (range 8.52-31.55), 16.1 kg/capita/year (range 2.32-29.88), respectively. With regard to egg consumption, Slovakia had the highest consumption and Poland the lowest. The United Kingdom had the highest poultry consumption and Croatia the lowest. Poland had the lowest bovine meat consumption and Luxembourg the highest. Regarding to climate, the median temperature in European countries was 11.4°C (range 1.68°C-19.85°C). Malta was the country with the highest median temperature and Finland with lowest media temperature. Median low temperature (1st percentile) was 2.38°C (range 1.95°C-13.69°C), and median high temperature (99th percentile) was 19.83°C (range 10.09°C-28.59°C). With respect to median low temperature, Finland was the lowest and Malta the highest. With respect to median high temperature, Iceland was the lowest and Cyprus the highest.

Socioeconomic indicators of the European countries are shown in Table 2. Median GDP per capita was 22,444 € (range 5,498 €-81,882 €) with very important differences; Luxembourg had the highest GDP and Bulgaria had the lowest. GINI index had a median of 30.2 (range 22.7-35.6). Iceland presented the lowest GINI index and Estonia the highest. Proportion of population in rural, urban cluster (towns) and high-density cluster (city) presented a median of 35% (range 0.2%-49.5%), 28.4% (range 9.7%-53.3%), and 38% (range 14.5%-89.5%), respectively. Malta was the country

Table 1. Characteristics of the European countries: Salmonellosis incidence, consumption of pork meat, bovine meat, poultry, and eggs, and temperatures median, low, and high

Country	Salmonella Infection[1]	Consumption[2]				Temperature °C[3]		
		Pork	Bovine	Poultry	Eggs	Median	Low	High
Austria	18.0	52.56	17.14	18.61	14.68	8.97	0.14	16.63
Belgium	23.4	38.65	15.63	12.20	12.59	12.63	4.6	19.31
Bulgaria	10.3	26.16	3.84	20.68	8,36	11.54	2.0	22.5
Croatia	35.2[4]	42.79	12.41	8.52	8.48	12.68	3.92	20.32
Cyprus	9.7	38.38	5.79	24.45	8.98	19.72	12.98	28.59
Czech Republic	109.6	41.17	8.15	19.09	11.66	10.91	0.40	19.92
Denmark	20.2	24.89	28.46	26.75	15.35	12.31	3.68	20.0
Estonia	10.5	29.68	7.19	21.11	12.66	6.24	-7.35	19.83
Finland	33.2	36.14	19.22	19.87	9.35	1.68	-11.95	17.99
France	28.3	33.05	23.81	22.93	13.85	13.05	7.23	18.46
Germany	21.3	51.81	13.16	17.75	12.2	12.02	2.04	19.81
Greece	3.5	28.31	16.10	15.74	10.73	13.84	7.27	24.5
Hungary	51.6	34.93	4.96	23.78	12.45	12.59	2.43	21.53
Iceland	13.6	26.87	13.36	26.87	8.24	1.77	-2.86	10.09
Italy	7.8 [5]	40.28	18.60	18.61	13.34	12.75	6.06	20.57
Latvia	16.5	34.96	5.11	20.53	14.03	7.21	-6.75	19.99
Lithuania	39.6	45.67	4.49	26.84	13.11	8.25	-5.96	20.24
Luxembourg	21.2	43.58	29.88	21.37	14.64	12.53	3.46	19.38
Malta	25.5	34.24	19.22	26.40	11.64	19.15	13.69	27.08
Netherlands	9.1	36.36	17.67	23.90	14.03	13.14	4.93	19.67
Norway	24.4	21.01	19.83	21.01	11.41	3.31	-5.25	15.31
Poland	20.2	46.19	2.32	27.41	7.53	10.2	-1.79	20.55
Portugal	2.1	37.91	16.45	30.14	9.05	16.45	8.94	22.25
Romania	7.1	25.31	4.78	15.38	12.94	10.61	0.27	20.57
Slovakia	72.8	31.78	5.19	15.13	16.05	10.3	0.39	19.41
Slovenia	22.2	28.19	18.19	23.46	9.36	11.40	2.33	18.51
Spain	40.0	48.92	12.15	28.63	13.32	14.38	6.53	22.67
Sweden	26.3	37.0	24.58	16.64	13.37	3.27	-9.63	17.29
United Kingdom	12.9	25.79	18.12	31.55	11.08	10.13	4.41	16.44
Ireland	6.4	26.26	22.35	26.26	8.96	10.08	5.11	15.96
Switzerland	15.4	31.49	21.26	16.38	10.53	9.27	0.46	14.77

1. Average salmonellosis incidence rate 2013-2014; 2. Consumption kg/capita/year, pork meat pork, bovine meat, poultry and eggs in 2013; 3. Temperature median range (1th -99th) percentiles 2014; 4. Croatia: Information 2013 year; 5. Italy: Information 2014 year.

Pork Meat Consumption and Salmonellosis Incidence ...

Table 2. Socioeconomic indicators.
European countries 2014-2015.

Country	GDP[1]/ 1000	GINI[2]	% Population[3]			% Population[4]		Physicians[5] 10⁵ inhab.	Health[6] Expend €
			Rural	Town	City	<5 y	< 15y		
Austria	36.37	27.6	40.7	29.4	29.8	4.7	14.3	509.7	4269
Belgium	33.83	25.9	18.0	53.2	28.8	5.8	17.0	301.8	3812
Bulgaria	5.50	35.4	34.2	26.4	39.5	4.7	13.7	404.5	518
Croatia	10.29	30.2	46.9	28.4	24.7	4.9	14.8	319.2	771
Cyprus	20.29	34.8	27.9	20.9	51.5	5.7	16.3	357.7	1408
Czech Republic	15.39	25.1	37.3	31.2	31.5	5.4	15.0	368.8	1157
Denmark	45.02	27.7	45.2	20.6	34.2	5.4	17.2	365.7	4938
Estonia	13.17	35.6	41.2	15.7	43.1	5.6	15.8	342.3	1003
Finland	34.22	25.6	30.1	35.7	34.2	5.6	16.4	320.6	3612
France	31.50	29.2	35.0	19.8	45.2	6.1	18.5	311.9	3623
Germany	34.09	30.7	23.2	41.4	35.4	4.2	13.2	413.9	4140
Greece	16.98	34.5	38.1	23.9	38.0	4.8	14.6	632.1	1361
Hungary	10.65	28.6	39.6	31.1	29.3	4.6	14.4	309.7	806
Iceland	33.99	22.7	14.9	20.5	64.7	7.1	20.5	377.6	3938
Italy	25.38	32.4	15.5	41.1	43.4	4.5	13.9	383.8	2437
Latvia	10.26	35.5	46.9	9.7	43.4	5.0	14.7	319.8	702
Lithuania	11.23	35.0	46.7	10.5	42.8	5.1	14.6	433.9	837
Luxembourg	81.88	28.7	48.9	36.6	14.5	5.7	16.8	290.7	5557
Malta	18.52	27.7	0.2	10.3	89.3	4.9	14.4	378.8	2449
Netherlands	38.67	26.2	14.7	40.2	45.1	5.3	16.9	347.5	4269
Norway	67.80	23.5	27.9	33.0	39.1	6.1	18.2	440.4	6697
Poland	10.63	30.8	42.3	24.5	33.2	5.2	15.0	232.8	718
Portugal	16.22	34.5	27.1	28.4	44.4	4.4	14.6	461.4	1555
Romania	6.97	35.0	49.5	17.8	32.8	4.8	15.5	276.6	400
Slovakia	13.60	26.1	41.3	35.1	23.6	5.4	15.3	345.1	999
Slovenia	17.54	25.0	44.8	36.4	18.8	5.3	14.6	282.5	1597
Spain	22.44	34.7	26.5	22.5	51.1	4.9	15.2	384.5	2123
Sweden	43.39	26.9	29.2	36.1	34.7	6.0	17.1	419.1	5023
United Kingdom	31.15	31.6	13.7	29.1	57.2	6.2	17.6	278.9	3938
Ireland	41.43	31.1	36.0	24.4	39.7	7.5	21.5	287.5	4273
Switzerland	57.47	32.9	-	-	74.1	5.1	14.8	411.0	7361

1. GDP = Gross Domestic Product per capita; 2. GINI index; 3.% Population: rural, town, city; 4.% Population under 5 years old, under 15 years old; 5. Per 10,000 inhabitants; 6. Healthcare expenditures per capita.

with the highest proportion of population in cities and Romania had the highest proportion of population in rural zones. With regard to the

88   *Alberto Arnedo-Pena and M. Rosario Pac-Sa*

proportion of the population under 5 years old and under 15 years old, a median was 5.3% (range 4.2%-7.5%) in the group under 5 years old and 15.2% (range 13.2%-21.5%) in the group under 15 years old. Germany had the lowest proportion of population under 5 and 15 years old, and Ireland the highest proportion of both 5 and 15 years old. In relation to physicians' density, the median was 357.7 per 100,000 inhabitants (range 232.8-632.1). Poland had the lowest physicians' density and Greece the highest. Median of healthcare expenditure was 2,437 € (range 400 €-7,361 €) with notable differences. Switzerland had the highest healthcare expenditure and Romania the lowest.

Analytic Approach

Spearman rank's correlations between salmonellosis incidence and all the explanatory variables estimated the grade of robustness and direction of the relationship (Table 3). The highest Spearman rank's correlations correspond to GINI index (-0.448) with inverse and significant relation to salmonellosis incidence (p = 0.012). Pork meat consumption presented a Spearman rank's correlation of 0.326 with a direct marginal significant association (p = 0.074). Proportion of population in cities, low temperature, and egg consumption shows lower Spearman rank's correlation, -0.321 (p = 0.098), -0.269 (p = 0.143) and 0.238 (p = 0.197), respectively.

In order to understand the relationship among explanatory variables, a Spearman rank's correlation was implemented for all these variables (Table 4). The following characteristics can be highlighted: first, bovine meat consumption had a direct association with GDP and healthcare expenditures and pork meat consumption was inversely associated with the proportion of population <15 years old. Second, poultry consumption was directly associated with the proportion of population in cities. Third, the proportion of rural population was inversely associated with GDP and healthcare expenditures. Fourth, GINI index presented an inverse association with the GDP, healthcare expenditures, and the proportions of population under 5 and 15 years old. Fifth, the GINI index was not associated with pork meat consumption or egg consumption, but it had an inverse association with bovine meat consumption.

Bivariate multilevel models of salmonellosis incidence with all explanatory variables are shown in Table 5. GINI index was significantly and inversely associated with salmonellosis (regression coefficient -2.55 and p = 0.001), and egg consumption presented a direct and significant association 3.12 (p = 0.039); pork meat consumption was marginally associated, regression coefficients 0.70 (p = 0.101). Bovine meat consumption had an inverse and weak association with salmonellosis (-0.79 p = 0.161). The remaining explanatory variables presented signification levels p $\geq$ 0.20.

Table 3. Spearman rank`s correlations coefficient between salmonellosis incidence and explanatory variables. European countries.

Variables	Coefficient	pvalue
Consumption: kg/capita/year		
Pork meat	0.326	0.074
Bovine meat	0.063	0.736
Poultry meat	-0.105	0.582
Eggs	0.238	0.197
Climate		
Temperature median	-0.117	0.531
Temperature low	-0.269	0.143
Temperature high	-0.093	0.617
Socio-economic indicators		
Gross Domestic Product per capita	-0.043	0.819
GINI index	-0.448	0.012
Rural population (%)	0.163	0.381
Town population (%)	0.140	0.462
City population (%)	-0.321	0.098
Population <5 years old (%)	0.106	0.369
Population <15 years old (%)	-0.014	0.941
Physicians per 100,000 inhabitants	-0.052	0.783

Table 4. Spearman rank´s correlation. Explanatory variables. European countries.

Variables	Food consumption				Population distribution			Population age-years		Socio-economic indicators			
	Po[1]	Bo[2]	Eg[3]	Po[4]	Rural	Town	City	<5 y	<15y	Gini	GDP[5]	Hc[6]	Phy[7]
Pork	-	0.20	0.16	-0.08	0.02	0.27	-0.12	-0.35	**-0.39**	0.04	0.04	-0.07	0.17
Bovine		-	0.20	0.05	-0.27	0.30	0.02	**0.40**	**0.42**	**-0.41**	*0.84*	*0.85*	0.09
Eggs			-	-0.17	0.21	0.10	-0.12	-0.04	0.04	-0.05	0.23	0.20	0.07
Poultry				-	0.20	**-0.36**	**0.57**	0.17	0.19	0.08	0.04	0.07	-0.11
Rural					-	0.25	*-0.55*	-0.10	-0.09	0.21	**-0.39**	**-0.44**	-0.30
Town						-	*-0.49*	-0.02	-0.16	*-0.53*	0.42	0.41	-0.01
City							-	0.12	0.16	0.29	-0.03	0.00	0.21
<5 years								-	*0.90*	**-0.39**	0.46	**0.44**	**-0.36**
<15 years									-	**-0.32**	**0.49**	**0.45**	-0.36
Gini index										-	*-0.48*	*-0.47*	0.09
GDP											-	*0.98*	0.20
Health-care												-	0.23
Physi-cians													-

1. Pork meat 2. Bovine meat 3. Eggs 4. Poultry 5. Gross Domestic Product per capita 6. Healthcare expenditure. 7. Physicians per 100,000 inhabitants.

Note: Bold type and cursive script indicate significant level $p < 0.05$, and $p < 0.01$, respectively.

A multivariate multilevel model of salmonellosis incidence is presented in Table 6. Only pork meat consumption and GINI index were associated with salmonellosis incidence. Salmonellosis rate increased by 0.79 (95% CI 0.11-1.48; p = 0.023) with the increment in pork meat consumption, adjusted by GINI index, -2.75 (95% CI -4.20 - -1.30; p = 0.000).The interclass correlation coefficient of the model was 0.31 (95% CI 0.04-0.83), this is, the proportion of the total variance of salmonellosis among countries that may be attributed region and climate levels. In addition, egg consumption was not found significantly associated with salmonellosis in a multivariate multilevel model, including pork meat consumption and GINI index, with a regression coefficient of 1.69 (95% CI -0.70-4.07 p = 0.165).

Table 5. Multilevel linear regression. Salmonellosis incidence and explanatory variables. Bivariate analysis. European countries.

Variables	Coefficient regression	95% Confidence Interval	pvalue
Consumption: kg/capita/year			
Pork meat	0.70	-0.10-1.56	0.101
Bovine meat	-0.69	-1.66- 0.28	0.161
Poultry meat	-0.51	-1.89-0.87	0.467
Eggs	3.12	0.16-6.09	0.039
Climate			
Temperature median	-0.16	-1.85-1.52	0.848
Temperature low	-0.36	-1.60-0.80	0.568
Temperature high	-0.17	-2.26-1.92	0.870
Socio-economic indicators			
Gross Domestic Product per capita	0.001	-0.47- 0.47	1.000
GINI index	-2.55	-4.11- -0.98	0.001
Rural population (%)	0.14	-0.51 - 0.79	0.680
Town population (%)	0.43	-0.30- 1.16	0.251
City population (%)	-0.24	-0.75- 0.27	0.355
Population< 5 years old (%)	0.76	-9.43- 10.83	0.883
Population < 15 years old (%)	-0.88	-4.86- 3.11	0.666
Physicians per 100,000 inhabitants	0.01	-0.11- 0.08	0.826
Healthcare expenditure per capita (euros)	0.002	-0.006- 0.002	0.318

The dose-response model between pork meat consumption and salmonellosis incidence is shown in Table 7. Three pork meat consumptions groups are contemplated 25th, 26-74th, and 75th percentiles, with 26.0 kg/capita/year 35.0 kg/capita/year and 45.9 kg/capita/year, respectively. The median of salmonellosis rates per 100,000 inhabitants of these three groups were 13.2, 16.5 and 28.3, respectively. The test for trend had a value of $z = 2.36$ (p = 0.018) in a bivariate analysis. A multilevel model considering the three groups adjusted for GINI index found higher salmonellosis rate when pork meat consumption increased. Considering reference 26 kg/capita/year, the regression coefficients of 26-74th and 75th percentiles were 13.8 (95% CI 0.93-26.60 p = 0.036) and 25.1 (95% CI 10.53-39.61 p = 0.001), respectively. In addition, the trend was significant (p = 0.001).

Table 6. Multilevel linear regression. Salmonellosis incidence and explanatory variables Multivariate analysis. European countries.

Variables	Regression coefficients	95% Confidence Interval	pvalue
Pork meat consumption[1]	0.79	0.11-1.48	0.023
GINI index	-2.75	-4.20- -1.30	0.000
Likelihood-ratio	Chi2 = 6.18	--	0.046
ICC[2]	0.31	0.04-0.83	
Goodness of fit			
	Null model	Present model	
Deviance	276.7284	263.6594	
Akaike's information criterion	284.7283	275.6593	
Bayesian information criterion	290.4643	284.2632	

1. Kg/capita/year 2. ICC = Interclass correlation coefficient.

Table 7. Pork meat consumption and salmonellosis incidence. Bivariate dose-response test for trend and multilevel linear regression. European countries.

Countries	Bivariate analysis		Multilevel analysis[1]		
	Pork meat[2] Median (range)	Salmonellosis[3] Median (range)	Regression coefficient	95% Confidence interval	pvalue
N = 8	26.0 (21.0-28.2)	13.2 (6.4-24.4)	Reference	-	
N = 15	35.0(28.3-40.3)	16.5 (2.5-72.9)	13.8	0.93-26.6	0.036
N = 8	45.9 (41.2-52.6)	28.3 (18-109.5)	25.1	10.5-39.6	0.001
LR[4]			Chi2 = 5.84		0.054
Trend[€]		0.018	Trend		0.001

1. Multilevel region and climate; adjusted for GINI index. 2. Consumption kg/capita/year. 3. Salmonellosis incidence rate.4. Likelihood-ratio

Countries with high pork meat consumption and high salmonellosis rate were Spain, Czech Republic, Lithuania, and Croatia, and the countries with a low salmonellosis rate and low pork meat consumptions Ireland, Romania, and Bulgaria. However, some countries like Austria and Germany presented elevated pork meat consumption and lower salmonellosis rate. In contrast, Slovakia and Hungary had high salmonellosis rates and low pork meat consumption.

DISCUSSION

The results of multilevel dose-response models suggested that pork meat consumption was associated with salmonellosis incidence. In addition, eggs and poultry consumptions were not significantly associated with salmonellosis incidence in the multilevel models. However, these results were not consistent for all countries. This could be explained due to the multiple factors associated with salmonellosis incidence. For instance, a recent research has estimated that eggs, pork, and poultry consumptions may cause 24%, 24%, and 20% of foodborne salmonellosis in Europe, respectively (Hoffman et al. 2017).

During the last years, the decrease of *S. Enteritidis salmonellosis* in European countries has been related to the reduction of contamination of eggs and poultry meat due to a significant improvement in hygiene in poultry farms through specific programs, and accurate information to the population (EFSA 2016). However, *S. Enteritidis* is still the *Salmonella* serovar more frequent, 44.4% of *Salmonella* serovars isolated in 2014, and 39.5% in 2015, versus 17.4% and 20.2% of *S. Typhimurium* in these years (EFSA 2015). In some European countries, an increase of salmonellosis by *S.* Typhimurium and other *Salmonella* serotypes, such as *S. Derby, S. Infantis, S. Rissen*, and *S. Goldcoast*, have been observed, and pork products consumption have been suggested as the vehicle of these salmonellosis (Andreoli et al. 2017, Simon et al. 2018, Schroeder et al. 2016, Garcia-Fierro et al. 2016, Scavia et al. 2013, Ronnqvist et al. 2018). *Salmonella* infections are transmitted and persist in pigs, and, interestingly, *Salmonella* serovars isolated in pigs are identical to isolated serovars in humans (Gymoese et al. 2017). *Salmonella* transmission mechanism in pigs is fecal-oral from infected pigs, but other mechanisms such as ingestion of contaminated feed or contact in abattoirs may be important. In general, one infected pig becomes a *Salmonella* asymptomatic carrier, and *Salmonella* is presented in tonsils, ileum, and intestinal epithelium; this carriage has no effect on pig growth (Van Parys et al. 2011). In four European countries a risk assessment model of salmonellosis due to pork consumption found that the risk of suffering salmonellosis ranges from 1 case per 100.000 to 10 per 10^6 serving,

94   *Alberto Arnedo-Pena and M. Rosario Pac-Sa*

considering pork cuts, mincemeat, and fermented ready-to-eat sausages; preparation at home and consumption had an elevated impact in the model (Vigre et al. 2016a, Swart et al. 2016).

Salmonella infections associated with pigs can be illustrated collecting information of human salmonellosis, *Salmonella* prevalence in swine farms and slaughterhouses, and *Salmonella* in pork products at retail establishments. In the last years, pork products consumption had been associated with salmonellosis foodborne outbreaks, which occurred in one European country, such as the United Kingdom, Spain, Germany, France, Denmark, and Italy (Paranthaman et al. 2013, de Frutos et al. 2018, Arnedo-Pena et al. 2016, Hernández-Arricibita et al. 2016, Schroeder et al. 2016, Gossner et al. 2012, Kuhn et al. 2013, Lettini et al. 2014), or in several countries, such as Denmark, Norway, and Sweden (Bruun et al, 2009), or Hungary and Italy (Coulombier and Takkinen 2013). In addition, sporadic cases of salmonellosis had been associated with pork products consumption in Hungary, Italy, Germany and Spain (Horváth et al. 2013, Scavia et al. 2013, Ziehm et al. 2013, Ziehm et al. 2015, Rettenbacher-Riefler et al. 2015, Arnedo-Pena et al. 2018). The systematic study of the prevalence of *Salmonella* in pigs took place in the 1990s in Denmark (Wegener et al. 2003), and in 2001-2003 in Germany (Merle et al. 2011). During the 2006-2007 period in European countries, the prevalence of *Salmonella* spp, *S.* Typhimurium, and *S.* Derby in positive lymph node sample in slaughter-pigs was 10.3%, 4.7%, and 2.1%, respectively, with maxim ranges of 29% (Spain), 16.1% (Luxembourg), and 6.5% (France), for *Salmonella* spp; and 0% in Finland (EFSA Journal 2008). In 2008, a European survey of EFSA (2009) *Salmonella* prevalence in breeding holdings was 28.1% and production holdings 29.0% with considerable variations among countries; in countries with more of 100 samples, the highest breeding holding prevalence was found in Spain (64.0%) and the lowest in Poland (6.9%); in production holdings, the highest prevalence was found in the Netherlands (55.7%) and the lowest in Finland (0.0%). In 2014, EFSA (2015) reported a *Salmonella* prevalence of 7.9% of pigs from farms or slaughterhouses in 11 European countries with bacteriological monitoring programs; the highest prevalence was observed in Denmark (21.6%) and Estonia (11.9%), whereas there was

0% prevalence in Norway and Sweden. In herd pigs, *Salmonella* prevalence was estimated to be 10.1%. In pigs, 54.7% *Salmonella* isolates were *S.* Typhimurium, and 17.5% *S.* Derby. Monophasic strains of *S.* Typhimurium represented 8.4% of the isolates. The monophasic strains are considered as potential epidemic due to high virulence and antibiotic resistances (Bone et al. 2010, Hauser et al. 2010, Bonardi 2017). Recent European studies of *Salmonella* prevalence in swine farms have found notable variation, such as in Spain 31% (Vico et al. 2011), Poland 30.0% (Dors et al. 2015), England 19.5% (Wales et al. 2013), and Germany 19.4% (Niemann et al. 2016).

Following pork production chain from farm to consumption, pigs are transported and slaughtered in abattoirs, and high prevalence of *Salmonella* is frequently detected in these places (Argüello et al. 2013), as it is found in different European studies as such by Powell et al. (2016) in England 30.5%, Piras et al. (2104) in Italy 15.9%, and De Brusser et al. (2011) in Belgium 14.1%. Some studies in Europe detected *Salmonella* in 7% of pork meat in Italy (Carraturo et al. 2016), 23.1% of pork meat from production units and retail markets in Romania (Mihaiu et al. 2014), 4,2% of fresh pork cuttings in Denmark (Hansen et al. 2010), and 2.6% of retail pork in Ireland (Prendergast et al. 2009). However, in a report of 2014 from EFAS (2015), proportions of pig products positive *Salmonella* in Europa were lower: 0.5% positive from 68,134 units of fresh pig meat at the slaughterhouse, and 0.7% positive from 20,259 samples of ready-to-eat minced meat, meat preparation, and meat products. *S.* Typhimurium was the most frequent serovar in pig meat (27.8%), followed by *S.* Derby (24.4%), and monophasic strains of *S.* Typhimurium (18%). In general, these studies support the hypothesis that pork meat consumption is associated with salmonellosis incidence.

With the objective of testing the validity of our results, three approaches were studied. First, a new multilevel model was made, considering a cluster with four groups of European countries according to their types of pork production (pig farms and slaughterhouses) and consumption (pork meat and sausages) following Vigre and co-authors research (Vigre et al. 2016b). In our model three levels were included, region, climate, and the cluster of four groups of European countries. Salmonellosis incidence presented a marginally significant association with pork meat consumption (0.68 95% CI -0.03-1.33 p = 0.068) adjusted by GINI index, and an interclass correlation coefficient of 0.69 (95% CI 0.30-0.92). Second, salmonellosis incidence in the 2013 year was studied by multilevel models. This incidence was significantly associated with pork meat consumption, coefficient 0.70 (95% CI 0.07-1.33 p = 0.028), adjusted for GINI index and an interclass correlation coefficient of 0.32 (0.04-0.83), with similar results with salmonellosis incidence 2013-2014 average. Finally, an underreporting factor of salmonellosis, described by Havelaar and colleagues (2013), was used to carry out a revision of salmonellosis incidence rates. No significant associated factors were found in multilevel analysis, including pork meat consumption and GINI index. This study of underreporting corresponds to the period 2005-2009, and it was made before the increase of salmonellosis associated with pork products. On the other hand, when underreporting of salmonellosis was included as an independent variable in multilevel models, salmonellosis incidence maintained the significant association with pork meat consumption (coefficient 0.74 95% CI 0.03-1.46 p = 0.043), adjusted by GINI index and an interclass correlation coefficient of 0.31 (95% CI 0.04-0.83).

In order to better understands which factors may be associated with this underreporting of salmonellosis, a Spearman rank`s correlations between underreporting and all explanatory variables were implemented (Table 8). Salmonellosis underreporting was directly associated with GINI index, temperature media, low and high. Inverse associations were found with GDP, healthcare expenditures, bovine meat consumption, proportion of population in town, and proportion of population less 5 years and 15 years old. In addition, the average of salmonellosis incidence rate was not associated with the underreporting (Spearman`s coefficient -0.27 p = 0.164). These results suggest that the GINI index inverse association with incidence of salmonellosis may be related to salmonellosis diagnostic and surveillance deficiencies as well as high salmonellosis incidence associated with insufficient hygiene practices in production and consumption of pork products; this took place in a context of low GDP and healthcare expenditures (Quinlan 2013). In multivariate multilevel models, the inclusion of GINI index may be adequate because other socio-economic indicators like GDP, healthcare expenditures were not associated with salmonellosis incidence.

Table 8. Spearman rank`s correlations coefficient between underreporting of salmonellosis (Havelaar 2013) and explanatory variables. European countries.

Variables	coefficients	pvalue
Consumption: kg/capita/year		
Pork meat	0.07	0.718
Bovine meat	-0.61	0.000
Poultry meat	0.17	0.374
Eggs	-0.24	0.212
Weather °C		
Temperature median	0.56	0.002
Temperature low	0.41	0.028
Temperature high	0.84	0.000
Socio-economic indicators		
Gross Domestic Product per capita	-0.75	0.000
GINI index	0.54	0.003
Rural population (%)	0.06	0.728
Town population (%)	-0.43	0.021
City population (%)	0.32	0.087
Population <5 years old (%)	-0.64	0.000
Population <15 years old (%)	-0.59	0.001
Physicians per 100,000 inhabitants	-0.12	0.521
Healthcare expenditure by inhabitant (euros)	-0.74	0.000

Strengths of this study reside in the following considerations: first, use of salmonellosis laboratory confirmed cases with the same case definition for all participant countries obtained from public European sources, EFSA and ECDCP. Second, data from independent variables were taken from different international sources, including FAOSTAT, EUROSTAT, and World Bank group. Third, proposed multilevel models were more robust than the classic multivariate linear regression. Fourth, multilevel analysis had permitted to adjust for different variables, obtaining more accurate results in a context with significant differences among European countries.

Fifth, demographic, socio-economic, and climatic differences in combination with food consumptions were studied, and significant associations were found like salmonellosis incidence and pork meat consumption adjusted for GINI index; on the other hand, in a study no significant association between the cluster of four groups of European countries and salmonellosis incidence was found (Vigre et al. 2016b). Our study highlights the importance of pork products in salmonellosis incidence apart that eggs consumption risk, but it has limitations.

Limitations of this study include the following: first, an ecological approach performs aggregate and average data of the population. The probability of occurrence of an ecological "fallacy" may be real if data are not representative of the population, distributions are skewed, and potential confusion factors and other variables are not studied. Second, there are considerable differences in the surveillance of salmonellosis in European countries, and several studies have indicated the magnitude of salmonellosis underreporting in some countries (Haagsma et al. 2013 Gibbons et al. 2014, Sadkowska-Todys and Czarkowski 2014, Mellou et al. 2013, Mølbak et al. 2014). Considering the year 2009, Havelaar and colleagues (2013) estimated a measure of this underreporting for European countries from information about returning Swedish travelers who suffer salmonellosis in Europe. This underreporting factor had a median of 28.9 (Czech Republic) with a range of 0.4 (Finland) and 2080 (Portugal). Six countries had an underreporting of more than 200.0 (Bulgaria, Greece, Malta, Romania, Spain, and Portugal) and three countries less than 2.0 (Sweden, Norway, and Finland). In general, a good surveillance together with the possibility of microbiologic confirmation may increase case-detection and reporting versus a more deficient surveillance. Third, *Salmonella* serotypes were not indicated in ECDPC and EFSA data, and transmission chains are conditioned by *Salmonella* serotypes reservoirs as well as poultry, swine, cattle, and it could generate some imprecision in our hypothesis (Simon et al. 2018). Fourth, *Salmonella* foodborne outbreaks may have effects in the reporting of cases and produce a bias on salmonellosis rate. Fifth, the analysis did not include some variables, such as specific control programs of *Salmonella* in swine farms, sausage consumption, or other unknown risk factors (Shaw et al.

2016). Sixth, some salmonellosis cases could be due to international travel and it may cause some misclassification of exposition. Seventh, four climate zone approach may be a simplification of climate variability in European countries.

In Europe, pork meat production and consumption have substantial differences. In 2014, considering pork meat production per capita, four countries (Denmark, Netherlands, Spain, and Germany) presented the highest productions: 283.3 kg/capita, 81.5 kg/capita, 77.5 kg/capita, 68.2 kg/capita, respectively. Countries with the highest production were Germany, Spain, and France with 5,507,000 tons, 3,620,220 tons, and 2,157,890 tons, respectively. On the other hand, four countries produce less than 10 kg per capita: Slovakia, Bulgaria, Slovenia, and Greece (EUROSTAT 2018). In European countries, there have been established four basic groups in the production and consumption of pork products (Vigre et al. 2016b), considering the size of pig farms and slaughters and consumption of pork meat and sausages. The first group with large farms and slaughters, and medium consumption of pork products includes Germany, Spain, Belgium, United Kingdom, Italy, France, Portugal, the Netherlands, Ireland, Cyprus, Denmark, and Sweden. The second group with small farms and slaughters, and medium consumption of pork products corresponds to Bulgaria, Hungary, Lithuania, Poland, Romania, and Slovenia. The third group with small farms and slaughters, and high consumption of pork products includes the Czech Republic, Estonia, Finland, Greece, Luxembourg, Latvia, Malta, and Slovakia. The fourth group includes Austria with small farms and large slaughters, and high consumption of pork meat but low of sausages.

In the European pig sector, *Salmonella* infections are well-known, and different interventions against these infections are carried out by European institutions and countries themselves. The European Union by different agencies, including ECDC and EFSA, has studied to know *Salmonella* prevalence in animals, food, and salmonellosis risk in humans, and has promulgated regulations and recommendations to avoid and prevent *Salmonella* food infections (EFSA 2018). These actions had considerable success against *Salmonella* in eggs and poultry, but with regard to

100 *Alberto Arnedo-Pena and M. Rosario Pac-Sa*

Salmonella infections in pigs no joint initiatives in the European Union have been implemented (Mainar-Jaime 2017). Economic recession, pork production complexity, complicated *Salmonella* epidemiology, and negative results of two cost-benefit analysis have blocked the compulsory implementation of *Salmonella* pig control programs (Argüello et al. 2017). In 2010, a study of the European Commission (2010) estimated in 90 million € the economic losses of human salmonellosis by pigs, but the cost-benefit analysis of implementing a program for the reduction of *Salmonella* in slaughter pigs suggested no economic benefit. A similar result of other cost-benefit analysis for the reduction of *Salmonella* in breeding pigs was published (European Commission 2011). It has been indicated a lack of precise data and information in some aspect of *Salmonella* infection on both pigs and humans, and this could be associated with failures of some studies (European Commission 2010). In the European Union regulations against *Salmonella* infections in pigs need to be carried out by national states, and regulations with high costs of implementation became difficult to address for European countries with low resources; in a free-border marker, this situation derives in a social and politic issue (Evangelopoulou et al. 2015).

In this context, few European countries have specific national programs against salmonellosis in the farm-to-consumption pork products chain. These countries include Norway, Finland, Sweden, and Denmark with a long tradition in control programs and others, such as the United Kingdom (Marier et al. 2016), Germany, Italy, Ireland (Argüello 2013) and Belgium (Méroc et al. 2012). In contrast, Eastern European countries do not have these national programs due to the high cost of implementation. In general, these programs estimate *Salmonella* prevalence in slaughter pig herd, and pig slaughter is done in function to detect risk (Wegener et al. 2003). In addition, biosecurity measures are required to prevent and reduce *Salmonella* infections in swine farms (Andres and Davies 2015), and other measures in the pork production and consumption chain are required (Snary et al. 2016). However, a part of the Scandinavian countries and Denmark, the effects of these programs in the reduction of *Salmonella* infection in pigs or humans have been controversial (Blaha 2018), and a new approach has been proposed in order to diminish *Salmonella* in pig slaughtered (Mainar-

Jaime et al. 2018). On the other hand, a lack of European regulations for specific control actions on pig farms associated with reiterated salmonellosis foodborne outbreaks has been pointed out in Germany, after two large outbreaks related to a primary production farm (Schielke et al. 2017).

Therefore, the pig sector in European countries offers considerable complexity, considering large differences in farms and abattoirs, pork production, and national variations in the consumption of pork products. Then, *Salmonella* infections control and prevention present special difficulty in their applications on the different countries, and it may be appropriate to know the specific conditions of each country. In this sense, some points can be highlighted, first, the implementation of national programs on *Salmonella* control in pig farms with the help and assistance of the European Union; second, increase public knowledge on *Salmonella* infections and pork products; third improve salmonellosis surveillance in many European countries.

CONCLUSION

This study suggests that pork meat consumption is associated with salmonellosis incidence in European countries. In the farm-to-consumption pork products chain, an increment and optimization of control and prevention measures are recommended.

REFERENCES

Alt K, Simon S, Helmeke C, Kohlstock C, Prager R, Tietze E, et al. Outbreak of uncommon O4 non-agglutinating *Salmonella* Typhimurium linked to minced pork, Saxony-Anhalt, Germany, January to April 2013. *PLoS One*. 2015;10:e0128349.

Andreoli G, Merla C, Valle CD, Corpus F, Morganti M, D'incau M, et al. Foodborne salmonellosis in Italy: characterization of *Salmonella* enterica serovar Typhimurium and monophasic variant 4,[5],12:i- isolated from salami and human patients. *J Food Prot.* 2017;80:632-639.

Andres VM, Davies RH. Biosecurity measures to control *Salmonella* and other infectious agents in pig farms: A Review. *Compr Rev Food Sci Food Saf 2015*;4:317-335.

Argüello H. *Swine salmonellosis in Spain: Risk factors in breeders, control strategies in the fattening stage and the importance of the slaughter.* Doctoral thesis, Leon University, Spain, 2013].

Argüello H, Alvarez-Ordoñez A, Carvajal A, Rubio P, Prieto M. Role of slaughtering in *Salmonella* spreading and control in pork production. *J Food Prot* 2013;76:899–911.

Argüello H, Carvajal A, Rubio P. *Pig health: Update on Salmonella control programs.* www.pig333.com/articles.2017 Accessed June 30, 2018.

Arnedo-Pena A, Vivas-Fornas I, Meseguer-Ferrer N, Tirado-Balaguer MD, Yagüe-Muñoz A, Herrera-León S, et al. Comparison of sporadic cases of *Salmonella* Typhimurium with other *Salmonella* serotypes in Castellon (Spain): case-case study. *Enferm Infecc Microbiol Clin.* 2018; 36:478-483.

Arnedo-Pena A, Bellido-Blasco JB, Romeu-Garcia MA, Meseguer-Ferrer N. Detection of foodborne *Salmonella* Typhimurium outbreaks. *Enferm Infecc Microbiol Clin.* 2017;35:470-471.

Arnedo-Pena A, Sabater-Vidal S, Herrera-León S, Bellido-Blasco JB, Silvestre-Silvestre E, Meseguer-Ferrer N, et al. An outbreak of monophasic and biphasic *Salmonella* Typhimurium, and Salmonella Derby associated with the consumption of dried pork sausage in Castellon (Spain). *Enferm Infecc Microbiol Clin.* 2016;34:544-550.

Blaha T. *The German Salmonella serological monitoring programme.* www.pig333.com/articles.2017 Accessed June 16, 2018.

Bonardi S. *Salmonella* in the pork production chain and its impact on human health in the European Union. *Epidemiol Infect.* 2017;145:1513-1526.

Bone A, Noel H, Le Hello S, Pihier N, Danan C, Raguenaud ME, et al. Nationwide outbreak of *Salmonella* enterica serotype 4,12:i:- infections in France, linked to dried pork sausage, March-May 2010. *Euro Surveill.* 2010;15: pii 19592.

Bruun T, Sørensen G, Forshell LP, Jensen T, Nygard K, Kapperud G, et al. An outbreak of *Salmonella* Typhimurium infections in Denmark, Norway and Sweden, 2008. *Euro Surveill.* 2009;14: pii19147.

Carraturo F, Gargiulo G, Giorgio A, Aliberti F, Guida M. Prevalence, Distribution, and diversity of *Salmonella* spp. in meat samples collected from Italian slaughterhouses. *J Food Sci.* 2016; 81:M2545-M2551.

Coulombier D, Takkinen J. From national to international--challenges in cross-border multi-country, multi-vehicle foodborne outbreak investigations. *Euro Surveill.* 2013;18:20423.

De Busser EV, Maes D, Houf K, Dewulf J, Imberechts H, De Zutter Lm et al. Detection and characterization of *Salmonella i*n lairage, on pig carcasses and intestines in five slaughterhouses. *Int J Food Microbiol.* 2011;145:279-86.

de Frutos M, López-Urrutia L, Berbel C, Allue M, Herrera S, Azcona JM, et al. Monophasic *Salmonella* Typhimurium outbreak due to the consumption of roast pork meat. *Rev Esp Quimioter.* 2018;31:156-159.

De Knegt LV, Pires SM, Hald T. Attributing foodborne salmonellosis in humans to animal reservoirs in the European Union using a multi-country stochastic model. *Epidemiol Infect* 2015;143:1175–1186.

Domínguez A, Torner N, Ruiz L, Martínez A, Bartolomé R, Sulleiro E, et al. Foodborne Salmonella-caused outbreaks in Catalonia (Spain), 1990 to 2003. *J Food Prot.* 2007;70:209-13.

Dors A, Pomorska-Mól M, Czyżewska E, Wasyl D, Pejsak Z. Prevalence and risk factors for Lawsonia intracellularis, Brachyspira hyodysenteriae and Salmonella spp. in finishing pigs in Polish farrow-to-finish swine herds. *Pol J Vet Sci.* 2015;18:825-31.

European Center of Disease Control and Prevention. Salmonellosis - Annual Epidemiological Report 2016 [2014 data]. *Annual Epidemiological Report on communicable diseases in Europe.* https://ecdc.europa.eu/en/publications-data/. Accessed April 14, 2018.

European Commission, European Office of Statistic. *EUROSTAT: Demographic, pork productions,* information http://appsso.eurostat.ec.europa.eu. Accessed May 22, 208.

European Commission. Analysis of the costs and benefits of setting a target for the reduction of Salmonella in slaughter pigs. *Food Control Consultans Consortium.* Health and Consumers Directorate-General Sanco/2008/E2/036 final report June 2010.

European Commission. Analysis of the costs and benefits of setting a target for the reduction of Salmonella in breeding pigs. *Food Control Consultans Consortium.* Health and Consumers Directorate-General. Sanco/2008/E2/036 final report March 2011.

European Food Safety Authority. Analysis of the baseline survey on the prevalence of Salmonella in holdings with breeding pigs, in the EU, 2008.Part A: *Salmonella* prevalence estimates. *EFSA Journal* 2009; 7:1377.

European Food Safety Authority. Panel on Biological Hazards (BIOHAZ). Scientific Opinion on monitoring and assessment of the public health risk of "*Salmonella* Typhimurium-like" strains. *EFSA Journal* 2010;8:1826.

European Food Safety Authority (EFSA) and European Centre for Disease Prevention and Control (ECDC). The European Union summary report on trends and sources of zoonoses, zoonotic agents and food-borne outbreaks in 2014. *EFSA Journal* 2015;13:4329.

European Food Safety Authority. The European Union summary report on trends and sources of zoonoses, zoonotic agents and food-borne outbreaks in 2016. *EFSA Journal* 2017;12:e05077.

European Food Safety Authority. Report of the Task Force on Zoonoses Data Collection on the analysis of the baseline survey on the prevalence of Salmonella in slaughter pigs, in the EU, 2006-20071 Part A: Salmonella prevalence estimates. *EFSA Journal* 2008; 135:1-111.

European Food Safety Authority. *Salmonella. What is Salmonella? How can we control and reduce it.* www.efsa.europa.eu/en/topics/topic/salmonella. Accessed June 6, 2018.

Evangelopoulou G, S. Kritas, G. Christodoulopoulos, A. R. Burriel. The commercial impact of pig *Salmonella* spp. infections in border-free markets during an economic recession. *Vet World.* 2015; 8: 257–272.

Foley SL, Lynne AM, Nayak R. *Salmonella* challenges: prevalence in swine and poultry and potential pathogenicity of such isolates. *J Anim Sci.* 2008;86(14 Suppl):E149-62.

Food Agriculture Organization (FAO). *United Nations.* http://www.fao.org/faostat/en/#data.Wed visited June 6, 2018.

Garcia-Fierro R, Montero I, Bances M, González-Hevia MÁ, Rodicio MR. Antimicrobial drug resistance and molecular typing of *Salmonella* enterica Serovar Rissen from different sources. *Microb Drug Resist.* 2016;22:211-7.

Gibbons CL, Mangen MJ, Plass D, Havelaar AH, Brooke RJ, Kramarz P, et al. Burden of communicable diseases in Europe (BCoDE) consortium. Measuring underreporting and under-ascertainment in infectious disease datasets: a comparison of methods. *BMC Public Health* 2014;14:147.

Gossner CM, van Cauteren D, Le Hello S, Weill FX, Terrien E, Tessier S, et al. Nationwide outbreak of *Salmonella* enterica serotype 4,[5],12:i:- infection associated with consumption of dried pork sausage, France, November to December 2011. *Euro Surveill.* 2012; 17: pii 20071.

Gymoese P, Sørensen G, Litrup E, Olsen JE, Nielsen EM, Torpdahl M. Investigation of outbreaks of *Salmonella* enterica Serovar Typhimurium and its monophasic variants using Whole-Genome Sequencing, Denmark. *Emerg Infect Dis.* 2017;23:1631-1639.

Haagsma JA, Geenen PL, Ethelberg S, Fetsch A, Hansdotter F, Jansen A, et al. Community incidence of pathogen-specific gastroenteritis: reconstructing the surveillance pyramid for seven pathogens in seven European Union member states. *Epidemiol Infect.* 2013;141:1625-39.

Hansen TB, Christensen BB, Aabo S. *Salmonella* in pork cuttings in supermarkets and butchers' shops in Denmark in 2002 and 2006. *Zoonoses Public Health.* 2010;57 Suppl 1:23-9.

Hauser E, Tietze E, Helmuth R, Junker E, Blank K, Prager R, et al. Pork contaminated with *Salmonella* enterica serovar 4,[5],12:i:-, an emerging health risk for humans. *Appl Environ Microbiol.* 2010; 76:4601-10.

Havelaar AH, Ivarsson S, Lofdahl M, Nauta MJ. Estimating the true incidence of campylobacteriosis and salmonellosis in the European Union, 2009. *Epidemiol Infect* 2013;13:1–10.

Hernández-Arricibita E, Santamaria-Zuazua R, Ramos-López G, Herrera-León S, Kárkamo- Zuñeda JA, Muniozguren-Agirre N.[Outbreak of *Salmonella* Typhimurium infections associated with consumption of chorizo in Bizkaia]. *Enferm Infecc Microbiol Clin.* 2016;34:577-578.

Hoffmann S, Devleesschauwer B, Aspinall W, Cooke R, Corrigan T, Havelaar A, et al. Attribution of global foodborne disease to specific foods: Findings from a World Health Organization structured expert elicitation. *PLoS One.* 2017; 12:e0183641.

Horváth JK, Mengel M, Krisztalovics K, Nogrady N, Pászti J, Lenglet A, et al. Investigation into an unusual increase of human cases of *Salmonella* Goldcoast infection in Hungary in 2009. *Euro Surveill.* 2013;18:20422.

Kovats RS, Edwards SJ, Hajati S, Armstrong BG, Ebi KL, Menne B. The effect of temperature on food poisoning: a time-series analysis of salmonellosis in ten European countries. *Epidemiol Infect* 2004;132:443–453.

Kuhn KG, Sørensen G, Torpdahl M, Kjeldsen MK, Jensen T, Gubbels S, et al. A long-lasting outbreak of *Salmonella* Typhimurium U323 associated with several pork products, Denmark, 2010. *Epidemiol Infect.* 2013;141:260-8.

Lake IR. Food-borne disease and climate change in the United Kingdom. *Environ Health.* 2017;16(Suppl 1):117.

Lettini AA, Saccardin C, Ramon E, Longo A, Cortini E, Dalla Pozza MC, et al. Characterization of an unusual *Salmonella* phage type DT7a and report of a foodborne outbreak of salmonellosis. *Int J Food Microbiol.* 2014;189:11-7.

Mainar-Jaime RC. *Other alternatives for the control of salmonella in pigs?* www.pig333.com/articles.2017 Accessed June 16, 2018.

Mainar-Jaime RC, Casanova-Higes A, Andrés-Barranco S, Vico JP. Looking for new approaches for the use of serology in the context of control programmes against pig salmonellosis. *Zoonoses Public Health.* 2018;65:e222–e228.

Marier E, Piers Smith R, Ellis-Iversen J, Watson E, Armstrong D, Hogeveen H, et al. Changes in perceptions and motivators that influence the implementation of on-farm Salmonella control measures by pig farmers in England. *Prev Vet Med.* 2016; 133:22-30.

Mellou K, Sideroglou T, Kallimani A, Potamiti-Komi M, Pervanidou D, Lillakou E, et al. Evaluation of underreporting of salmonellosis and shigellosis hospitalized cases in Greece, 2011: results of a capture-recapture study and a hospital registry review. *BMC Public Health.* 2013;13:875.

Merle R, Kösters S, May T, Portsch U, Blaha T, Kreienbrock L. Serological *Salmonella* monitoring in German pig herds: results of the years 2003-2008. *Prev Vet Med.* 2011;99:229-33.

Méroc E, Strubbe M, Vangroenweghe F, Czaplicki G, Vermeersch K, Hooyberghs J, et al. Evaluation of the *Salmonella* surveillance program in Belgian pig farms. *Prev Vet Med.* 2012;105:309-14.

Mihaiu L, Lapusan A, Tanasuica R, Sobolu R, Mihaiu R, Oniga O, et al. First study of *Salmonella* in meat in Romania. *J Infect Dev Ctries.* 2014;8:50-8.

Mølbak K, Simonsen J, Jørgensen CS, Krogfelt KA, Falkenhorst G, Ethelberg S, et al. Seroincidence of human infections with nontyphoid *Salmonella* compared with data from public health surveillance and food animals in 13 European countries. *Clin Infect Dis.* 2014;59:1599-606.

Mughini-Gras L, Enserink R, Friesema I, Heck M, van Duynhoven Y, van Pelt W. Risk factors for human salmonellosis originating from pigs, cattle, broiler chickens and egg laying hens: a combined case-control and source attribution analysis. *PLoS One.* 2014;9:e87933.

Niemann JK, Alter T, Gölz G, Tietze E, Fruth A, Rabsch W, et al. Simultaneous occurrence of *Salmonella* enterica, *Campylobacter* spp. and *Yersinia* enterocolitica along the pork production chain from farm to meat processing in five conventional fattening pig herds in Lower Saxony. *Berl Munch Tierarztl Wochenschr.* 2016; 129:296-303.

Omer MK, Álvarez-Ordoñez A, Prieto M, Skjerve E, Asehun T, Alvseike OA. Systematic review of bacterial foodborne outbreaks related to red meat and meat products. *Foodborne Pathog Dis.* 2018 Jun 29. doi: 10.1089/fpd.2017.2393.

Parada J, Carranza A, Alvarez J, Pichel M, Tamiozzo P, Busso J, et al. Spatial distribution and risk factors associated with *Salmonella* enterica in pigs. *Epidemiol Infect.* 2017;145:568-574.

Paranthaman K, Haroon S, Latif S, Vinnyey N, de Souza V, Welfare W, et al. Emergence of a multidrug-resistant (ASSuTTm) strain of *Salmonella* enterica serovar Typhimurium DT120 in England in 2011 and the use of multiple-locus variable-number tandem-repeat analysis in supporting outbreak investigations. *Foodborne Pathog Dis.* 2013;10(10):850-5.

Piras F, Fois F, Mazza R, Putzolu M, Delogu ML, et al. *Salmonella* prevalence and microbiological contamination of pig carcasses and slaughterhouse environment. *Ital J Food Saf.* 2014;3:4581.

Powell LF, Cheney TE, Williamson S, Guy E, Smith RP, Davies RH. A prevalence study of *Salmonella* spp., *Yersinia* spp., *Toxoplasma* gondii and porcine reproductive and respiratory syndrome virus in UK pigs at slaughter. *Epidemiol Infect.* 2016;144:1538-49.

Prendergast DM, Duggan SJ, Gonzales-Barron U, Fanning S, Butler F, Cormican M, et al. Prevalence, numbers and characteristics of *Salmonella* spp. on Irish retail pork. *Int J Food Microbiol.* 2009; 131:233-9.

PVSITES. Consortium. European climate zones and bio-climatic design requirements. *Project Bear-iD, Nobatek 2016.* www.pvsites.eu. Wed visit June 7, 2018.

Quinlan JJ. Foodborne illness incidence rates and food safety risks for populations of low socioeconomic status and minority race/ethnicity: a review of the literature. *Int J Environ Res Public Health.* 2013;10:3634-52.

Rettenbacher-Riefler S, Ziehm D, Kreienbrock L, Campe A, Pulz M, Dreesman J. Sporadic salmonellosis in Lower Saxony, Germany, 2011-2013: raw ground pork consumption is associated with Salmonella Typhimurium infections and foreign travel with *Salmonella* Enteritidis infections. *Epidemiol Infect.* 2015; 143:2777-85.

Ronnqvist M, Valttil V, Ranta J, Tuominen P. *Salmonella* risk to consumers via pork is related to the Salmonella prevalence in pig feed. *Food Microbiol* 2018;71:93-97.

Sadkowska-Todys M, Czarkowski MP. Salmonellosis in Poland in 2012. *Przegl Epidemiol.* 2014;68:243-8, 353-5.

Scavia G, Ciaravino G, Luzzi I, Lenglet A, Ricci A, Barco L, et al. A multistate epidemic outbreak of *Salmonella* Goldcoast infection in humans, June 2009 to March 2010: the investigation in Italy. *Euro Surveill.* 2013;18:20424.

Schroeder S, Harries M, Prager R, Höfig A, Ahrens B, Hoffmann L, et al. A prolonged outbreak of *Salmonella* Infantis associated with pork products in central Germany, April-October 2013. *Epidemiol Infect.* 2016;144:1429-39.

Schielke A, Rabsch W, Prager R, Simon S, Fruth A, Helling R, et al. Two consecutive large outbreaks of *Salmonella* Muenchen linked to pig farming in Germany, 2013 to 2014: Is something missing in our regulatory framework? *Euro Surveill.* 2017;22; pii 30528.

Shaw KS, Cruz-Cano R, Jiang C, Malayil L, Blythe D, Ryan P, et al. Presence of animal feeding operations and community socioeconomic factors impact salmonellosis incidence rates: An ecological analysis using data from the Foodborne Diseases Active Surveillance Network (FoodNet), 2004-2010. *Environ Res.* 2016;150:166-72.

Silva C, Calva E, Maloy S. One health and food-borne disease: *Salmonella* transmission between humans, animals, and plants. *Microbiol Spectr.* 2014;2:OH-0020-2013.

Simon S, Trost E, Bender J, Fuchs S, Malorny B, Rabsch W, et al. Evaluation of WGS based approaches for investigating a food-borne outbreak caused by *Salmonella* enterica serovar Derby in Germany. *Food Microbiol.* 2018;71:46-54.

Smyth B, Evans DS, Kelly A, Cullen L, O'Donovan D. The farming population in Ireland: mortality trends during the 'Celtic Tiger' years. *Eur J Public Health.* 2013;23:50-5.

Snary EL, Swart AN, Simons RR, Domingues AR, Vigre H, Evers EG, et al. A quantitative microbiological risk assessment for *Salmonella* in pigs for the European Union. *Risk Analysis* 2016;36:437-449.

Swart AN, van Leusden F, Nauta MJ. A QMRA model for *Salmonella* in pork products during preparation and consumption. *Risk Analysis* 2016;36:516-530.

Van Parys A, Boyen F, Leyman B, Verbrugghe E, Haesebrouck F, Pasmans F. Tissue-specific *Salmonella* Typhimurium gene expression during persistence in pigs. *PLoS One.* 2011;6:e24120.

Vico JP, Rol I, Garrido V, San Román B, Grilló MJ, Mainar-Jaime RC. Salmonellosis in finishing pigs in Spain: prevalence, antimicrobial agent susceptibilities, and risk factor analysis. *J Food Prot.* 2011;74:1070-8.

Vigre H, Barfoed K, Swart AN, Simons RR, Hill AA, Snary EL, et al. Characterization of human risk of salmonellosis related to consumption of pork products in different E.U. Countries based on a QMRA. *Risk Analysis* 2016;36:531-545.(a)

Vigre H, Domingues AR, Pedersen UB, Hald T. An approach to cluster EU member states into groups according to pathways of *Salmonella* in the farm-to consumption chain for pork products. *Risk Analysis* 2016;36:450-460.(b).

Wegener HC, Hald T, Lo Fo Wong D, Madsen M, Korsgaard H, Bager F, et al. *Salmonella* control programs in Denmark. *Emerg Infect Dis.* 2003;9:774-80.

Wales A, Weaver J, McLaren IM, Smith RP, Mueller-Doblies D, Davies RH. Investigation of the distribution of *Salmonella* within an integrated pig preeding and production organisation in the United Kingdom. *ISRN Vet Sci.* 2013;2013:943126.

World Bank Group. *Climate change knowledge portal.* http://sdwebx. worldbank.org/climateportal. Accessed June 7, 2018.

Yang X, Jin K, Yang F, Yuan G, Liu W, Xiang L, et al. Nontyphoidal *Salmonella* gastroenteritis in Baoshan, Shanghai, China, 2010 to 2014. An etiological surveillance and case-control study. *J Food Prot.* 2017;80:482-487.

Ziehm D, Rettenbacher-Riefler S, Kreienbrock L, Campe A, Pulz M, Dreesman J. Risk factors associated with sporadic salmonellosis in children: a case-control study in Lower Saxony, Germany, 2008-2011. *Epidemiol Infect.* 2015;143:687-94

Ziehm D, Dreesman J, Campe A, Kreienbrock L, Pulz M. Risk factors associated with sporadic salmonellosis in adults: a case-control study. *Epidemiol Infect.* 2013;141:284-92.

INDEX

A

adipose tissue, 9, 23, 27
animals, vii, 1, 2, 5, 6, 9, 47, 48, 52, 53, 56, 57, 58, 59, 60, 66, 69, 71, 73, 99, 107, 109

B

brain, viii, 2, 8, 14, 16, 49, 52, 53, 57
by-products, 7, 8, 24, 25

C

calcium, vii, viii, 2, 9, 14, 16, 19, 30
climate, vii, ix, 54, 55, 80, 82, 83, 84, 85, 90, 92, 95, 99, 106, 108
cooked pork meat, vii, viii, 2, 19
cooking, viii, 2, 8, 18, 19, 20, 21, 22, 28, 33, 67
copper, vii, viii, 2, 9, 14, 17, 19

D

dose-response model, 91, 93

E

edible by-products, 7, 8
edible offal, viii, 2, 8, 9, 14, 16, 20, 23, 27, 35, 43
eggs consumption, 98
European Centre Disease Prevention and Control, 82
European Commission, 82, 100, 103, 104
European countries, vii, ix, 79, 80, 81, 82, 83, 84, 85, 86, 87, 89, 90, 91, 92, 93, 94, 95, 97, 98, 99, 100, 101, 106, 107
European Food Safety Authority, ix, 80, 82, 104

F

fancy meat, 8
fat, vii, 1, 6, 7, 8, 9, 11, 17, 22, 36, 42
fatty tissues, 7, 18
Food Agriculture Organization, 105

foodborne diseases, 80

G

GINI index, x, 80, 82, 85, 87, 88, 89, 90, 91, 92, 96, 97, 98

H

heart, viii, 2, 8, 14, 16, 18, 48, 53, 56, 57

I

incidence rate, ix, 80, 82, 84, 85, 86, 92, 96, 108, 109
internal organs, 7, 8
iron, vii, viii, 2, 3, 9, 14, 16, 19, 20

K

kidney, viii, 2, 3, 8, 9, 14, 16, 18, 23, 26, 27, 28, 36

L

lard, 18
leaf fat, 18
lipids, 9
liver, viii, 2, 8, 9, 14, 16, 18, 23, 25, 26, 28, 33, 50
lungs, viii, 2, 8, 14, 16, 18

M

macrominerals, viii, 2, 27, 38, 43
magnesium, vii, viii, 2, 9, 14, 16, 19, 20
manganese, vii, viii, 2, 9, 14, 17, 18, 19, 20
meat, vii, ix, 1, 6, 7, 8, 9, 17, 18, 19, 20, 22, 23, 24, 25, 26, 28, 29, 32, 33, 34, 37, 38,

39, 46, 47, 53, 56, 60, 62, 66, 74, 76, 77, 79, 80, 81, 82, 85, 86, 88, 89, 90, 91, 92, 93, 95, 96, 97, 99, 103, 107
Mexico, v, viii, 45, 46, 48, 51, 52, 54, 55, 56, 57, 58, 59, 60, 62, 64, 66, 67, 68, 69, 70, 71, 72, 73, 74, 77
microminerals, viii, 2, 27, 43
micronutrients, vii, 1, 6, 7
mineral retention, 20
minerals, vii, 1, 2, 3, 4, 5, 6, 8, 19
molecular detection, 46, 54, 76, 77
muscle tissue, 9, 61
muscles, vii, 1, 5, 9

N

nutritional quality, 6, 34

O

outbreaks, x, 57, 66, 67, 74, 80, 81, 84, 94, 98, 101, 102, 103, 104, 105, 107, 109

P

parasites, vii, viii, 45, 46, 47, 48, 50, 54, 56, 61, 65, 66, 67, 68, 69
phosphorous, vii, viii, 2, 9, 14, 19, 20
pig, viii, 2, 7, 8, 9, 16, 17, 18, 20, 22, 24, 25, 26, 27, 29, 34, 40, 46, 48, 49, 55, 56, 58, 59, 67, 72, 73, 76, 81, 82, 93, 95, 99, 100, 101, 102, 103, 104, 106, 107, 108, 109, 110
pig edible offal, viii, 2, 16, 18, 20
pig-meat, 46
pork, vii, viii, ix, 2, 6, 9, 10, 12, 14, 17, 18, 19, 20, 21, 22, 23, 24, 26, 27, 28, 29, 31, 32, 34, 35, 38, 41, 42, 43, 45, 46, 47, 48, 49, 53, 54, 55, 56, 57, 58, 60, 62, 64, 66, 67, 72, 75, 76, 77, 79, 80, 81, 82, 84, 85,

Index

86, 88, 89, 90, 91, 92, 93, 94, 95, 96, 98, 99, 100, 101, 102, 103, 105, 106, 107, 108, 109, 110

pork meat, viii, ix, 2, 9, 10, 12, 14, 17, 18, 19, 20, 48, 55, 72, 79, 80, 81, 82, 84, 85, 86, 88, 89, 90, 91, 92, 93, 95, 98, 99, 101, 103

pork meat consumption, ix, 80, 82, 84, 85, 88, 89, 90, 91, 92, 93, 95, 96, 98, 101

porkborne illnesses, vii, viii, 45, 46

potassium, vii, viii, 2, 9, 14, 19, 30

prevention, ix, x, 46, 48, 53, 67, 80, 101

R

raw pig edible offal, 14, 15, 16

red meat, 107

regions, 48, 54, 57, 60, 66

S

S. Typhimurium, ix, 79, 80, 81, 83, 93, 94, 95

Salmonella, x, 34, 80, 81, 84, 86, 93, 94, 95, 98, 99, 100, 101, 102, 103, 104, 105, 106, 107, 108, 109, 110

Salmonella Derby, 102

Salmonella Typhimurium, 101, 102, 103, 104, 106, 108, 110

Salmonellosis, v, vii, ix, 79, 80, 81, 82, 83, 84, 86, 88, 89, 90, 91, 92, 93, 94, 95, 96,

97, 98, 99, 100, 101, 102, 103, 105, 106, 107, 108, 109, 110, 111

Salmonellosis underreporting, 96

skeletal muscles, vii, 1, 6, 8, 9

sodium, vii, viii, 2, 3, 9, 14, 19, 20, 30, 38

Spearman rank's correlation, 84, 88

spinal cord, viii, 2, 8, 14, 16, 18

spleen, viii, 2, 8, 14, 16, 18

swine, ix, 47, 56, 63, 67, 72, 76, 77, 79, 80, 94, 98, 100, 103, 105

T

T. gondii, viii, 45, 46, 47, 52, 53, 54, 55, 56, 60, 62, 63, 64, 65, 66, 67

T. solium, viii, 45, 46, 48, 49, 51, 59, 66, 67

T. spiralis, viii, 45, 46, 57, 58, 60, 66, 67, 74

tongue, viii, 2, 8, 14, 16, 18, 53, 56, 59, 62, 75

V

variety meat, 8

Z

zinc, vii, viii, 2, 9, 14, 17, 19, 20

zoonosis, 46, 73, 80

Milk Consumption and Health

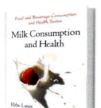

Editors: Ebbe Lange and Felix Vogel

Series: Food and Beverage Consumption and Health

Book Description: Milk proteins have a great potential use as functional foods. This book presents the views of some of the world's top nutrition scientists on this food that has served mankind for over 10,000 years.

Hardcover ISBN: 978-1-60741-459-9
Retail Price: $135

Garlic Consumption and Health

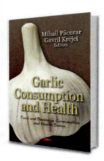

Editors: Mihail Păcurar and Gavril Krejci

Series: Food and Beverage Consumption and Health

Book Description: Despite the numerous therapeutic effects attributed to garlic, the chemistry behind its health-promoting effects is still poorly understood. This book attempts to address this problem, as well as the effects of garlic on cardiovascular diseases and the side effects that may develop from the consumption of garlic.

Hardcover ISBN: 978-1-60741-642-5
Retail Price: $265

Fish Consumption and Health

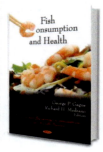

Editors: George P. Gagne and Richard H. Medrano

Series: Food and Beverage Consumption and Health

Book Description: This book presents current research on the benefits as well as the risks of fish consumption. The health benefits discussed include the reduction of cardiovascular disease, the decreased risk of various malignancies, specifically, colorectal, breast, prostate and lung cancers.

Hardcover ISBN: 978-1-60741-151-2
Retail Price: $135

Food Labelling: The FDA's Role in the Selection of Healthy Foods

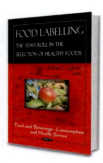

Editor: Ethan C. Lefevre

Series: Food and Beverage Consumption and Health

Book Description: The Food and Drug Administration (FDA) oversees federal labeling rules for 80 percent of foods. This book explores Food Labelling in the U.S., wherein the FDA needs to better leverage resources, improve oversight and effectively use available data to help consumers select healthy foods.

Softcover ISBN: 978-1-60692-898-1
Retail Price: $59